You don't have to be bored when you diet!

USE THE FINGERTIP LOW CALORIE GUIDE

CHAPTER 15

to find out which foods are
200-350 calories
100-200 calories
50-100 calories
20-50 calories
20 calories or less

You'll find delicious surprises like these...

Under 20 calories:
1 dill pickle
1 cup spinach

Under 50 calories:
1 egg roll
1 cup popcorn

Under 100 calories:
1 extra light beer
4 ounces gefilte fish

Under 200 calories:
7 ounces beef stew with biscuits
7½ ounces macaroni and cheese

Under 350 calories:
13 ounces eggplant parmigiana
8 ounces oysters

Also by
Bernard Le Gette

Le Gette's Guide To Fresh Food Shopping

Published by
WARNER BOOKS

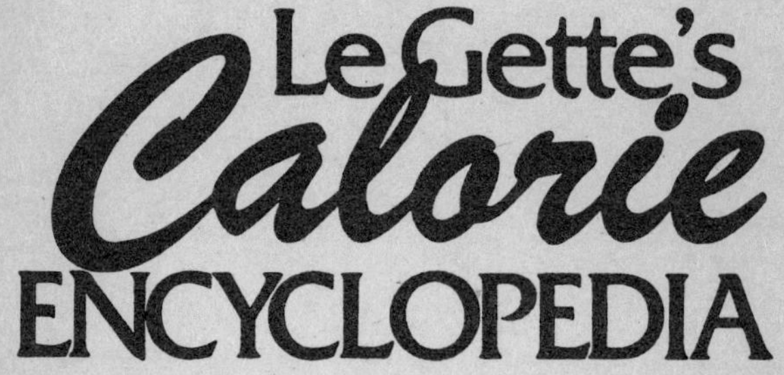

Bernard Le Gette

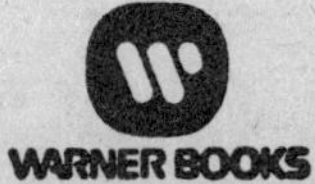

A Warner Communications Company

WARNER BOOKS EDITION

Cover photo by Frank Marchesano

Warner Books, Inc.
666 Fifth Avenue
New York, N.Y. 10103

A Warner Communications Company

Printed in the United States of America

First Printing: January, 1983

10 9

Contents

Introduction

Losing weight is simple. It's not easy—but it's simple. You cut the intake of your calories, and then you lose weight. Everything else you've ever heard is icing on the cake you can't eat. Carbohydrates, cholesterol, volume, protein, metabolism, exercise, are all very interesting, and confusing, to think about, though none of these things plays a big role in how much you weigh or how little you can weigh.

But even when people cut calories they usually don't do a very good job of it. You have probably gone on diets, wondered why they didn't work and wandered off them again, or maybe they did work, but your will power collapsed—

the constant pressure of not eating so many delicious foods caved you right in.

There are two reasons why most people fail. The first is that they don't really know how many calories they're consuming. They estimate how many calories are in each food, estimate how much of each food they ate, and constantly say things like, "That was only a little snack—two or three crackers." Sound familiar? And of course they're always rejecting potatoes.

Well I'll tell you right now, there is no way you can estimate. You can't estimate the size, you can't estimate the number of calories and you can't estimate the number of times you snacked. You can't estimate a thing. You aren't that smart. Nobody is.

You have to count the pieces, weigh them, and check every time how many calories you just ate. And then you have to write it down. Every calorie. Every day.

Now I know this is more inconvenient than being fat, and hating yourself every day, and being tired, and having heart attacks. But that's the way it is. It does have the advantage of being one inconvenience instead of many, and it is also only one simple way to lose weight—instead of many complicated ways not to—which brings us to the second reason most people fail.

It's because losing weight tends to get very vague in people's minds. It's a hidden enemy that has to be strained against every day. And that's very disheartening—which means it won't work. Any constant general restriction on your life, that has no definite limits and no clear procedure, is just not going to work. That's why specific diets are so successful in the short term—they remove the vagueness, the guesswork, the doubt. But we aren't talking about the short term. We're talking about weighing whatever you like for the rest of your life.

Fortunately, you don't have to fight hidden enemies. You don't even have to use much will power. You only have to know how to count—calories.

The purpose of this book and the years of research that went into it is to give you—in one place—the calories of all the foods you might ever eat. Whether it's fresh, or a commercially packaged brand, or a meal you ate in a restaurant or prepared at home, or a snack you ate at a drive-in—it's here. The portions listed are as standardized as is practical, so you don't have to bring your calculator. There are no extra columns of things that won't help you lose weight, and there is as little repetition as possible. You won't find listings of Thingamajigs—25 calories; Thingamajigs on a stick—25 calories; Thingamajigs sliced—25 calories, and so on. If thingamajigs are 25 calories, that's all you need to read—very simple.

The chapters are in a logical order chosen to

help you remember where things are listed. If everything were listed alphabetically you wouldn't know if some fish would be found under fillet, or haddock, or Mrs. Paul's, and even when you found it you couldn't compare it to others of its kind. So everything is in these fourteen basic groupings.

And the fifteenth chapter is the Fingertip Low Calorie Guide. This is an innovation which I hope will enable you to find a variety of low calorie foods at a glance. They are listed in calorie groups so you can plan your shopping, your meals, even your snacks with a specific number of calories in mind. It is also a pretty thorough list of the low calorie foods available. As you'll see in the rest of the book, being called *low calorie* or *dietetic* is no guarantee that a food is low in calories.

Everything is listed for normal usage. That is, if a food is made from a mix, say, the quantity and the calories listed are for the food after it's been prepared according to the package instructions. Likewise, it is of no use to know how many calories are in a pound of spinach while it is still frozen, so that is not listed. Now some things are listed as containing 0 calories for one tsp, and that is accurate; it is also reasonably accurate for one tbs. I can't guarantee, however, that there are no calories in three lbs. of sweetener. There just might be a few.

So how do you lose weight? Eat *what* you want, though of course a balanced diet is always best. It's not what, but *how many* that counts. Remember, virtually all foods have calories. The question is, how much satisfaction and/or nutrition are you getting from a particular food? For the calories in it, a plain potato contains a phenomenal variety of nutrients— you can probably live longer on potatoes than on any other single food—and that would suit some people fine. Others, however, would like to go quickly on apples, which contain neither calories nor nutrients in any marked degree.

But however you do it—eat fewer calories. Measure every portion. It's quite easy. Just put your chicken, or your potato, on a scale, see what the scale says, and compare that to the portion listed in this book. Write down the number of calories for each meal. Add them up at the end of the day, and in the morning write down how much you weigh next to yesterday's calorie total.

But you have to do it every time. It won't do you any good sometimes. And if after awhile you think you can remember most foods' calories, you're wrong. You have to measure. You have to count. The reason you're fat (which is why you bought this book) is you don't know how to play it by eye. You were brought up to eat too much, your aggression makes you hungry, your metabolism is rotten, whatever. It doesn't matter. You want to be thin. I just told you how. If you really *want* to be thin, that's what you'll do. Otherwise you'll continue to play at it and make excuses.

Now if you want to look good and be completely healthy *in addition* to being thin, you'll also exercise, though the exercise won't do either of those things for you if you're overweight. And it won't help you to lose much weight either. The relation between calories and exercise is straightforward. The harder it is, the more calories you burn. There are 3,600 calories in 1 pound of fat. Roughly, you'll burn 100 calories by:

skating (either kind)	45	minutes
skiing (either kind)	35	"
football	30	"
handball	22	"
walking	19	"
rowing	18	"
bicycling	15	"
chopping wood	13	"
swimming	12	"
jumping rope	11	"
jogging	10	"
running	6	"

or (even more roughly) 18 holes of golf (on foot) or two sets of tennis.

So if you want to lose that pound of fat, it's easier not to eat the 3,600 calories than to jump rope for 7 hours. What will help the most is a regular, steady approach to food and calories. This book can be your guide to help you look and feel the person you really want to be.

1 quart	**=**	**4 cups**
1 cup	**=**	**8 fluid ounces (oz)**
1 cup	**=**	**½ pint**
1 cup	**=**	**16 tablespoons**
1 ounce	**=**	**2 tablespoons**
1 tablespoon (tbs.)	**=**	**3 teaspoons**
1 jigger, or shot	**=**	**1½ ounces**
1 pound (lb.)	**=**	**16 ounces**

Remember, a fluid ounce is a measure of volume, not weight.

ALL listings are for food *as prepared* for normal usage. That means that after it's been prepared with all the normal ingredients, and it's ready to eat—that's what the calories are for.

CHAPTER 1

Beverages

SPIRITS, WINES, LIQUEURS, COCKTAILS, BRANDIES, AND COCKTAIL MIXES

Note: The number of calories in distilled spirits depends entirely on the alcoholic content—the higher the proof, the higher the calories. This is true for bourbon, gin, rum, Scotch, tequila, vodka, and almost anything called whiskey.

1

Distilled Spirits, 1 oz

80 proof	65
90 proof	75
100 proof	85
150 proof	125

Cocktails, canned or bottled, alcoholic, 1 oz

Amaretto Sour	
Mr. Boston	40
Apricot Sour	
Party Tyme	33
Banana Daiquiri	
Party Tyme	33
Daiquiri	
Hiram Walker	59
Mr. Boston	33
Party Tyme	33
Calvert	63
Gimlet	
Party Tyme	40
Gin & Tonic	
Party Tyme	28
Mai Tai	
Lemon Hart	60
Mr. Boston	36
Party Tyme	33

Manhattan	
Calvert	54
Mr. Boston	40
Party Tyme	37
Margarita	
Calvert	59
Mr. Boston	35
Mr. Boston strawberry	45
Party Tyme	33
Martini, Gin	
Calvert	63
Hiram Walker	55
Mr. Boston	33
Party Tyme	41
Martini, Vodka	
Calvert	63
Hiram Walker	49
Mr. Boston	34
Party Tyme	36
Old Fashioned	
Hiram Walker	55
Piña Colada	
Mr. Boston	60
Party Tyme	32
Rum & Cola	
Party Tyme	28
Screwdriver	
Mr. Boston	39
Party Tyme	35

Sour, Gin	
Calvert	65
Sour, Scotch	
Party Tyme	33
Sour, Tequila	
Calvert	65
Sour, Whiskey	
Calvert	60
Hiram Walker	60
Mr. Boston	40
Tequila Sunrise	
Mr. Boston	40
Tom Collins	
Calvert	65
Party Tyme	29
Vodka Tonic	
Party Tyme	27
Wallbanger	
Mr. Boston	34

Cocktail Mixes, bottled and dry, nonalcoholic, 1 oz or 1 premeasured packet

Alexander	
Holland House	69
Amaretto	
Holland House	79
Banana Daiquiri	
Holland House	66

Mint Julep	
Holland House	67
Old Fashioned	
Holland House	9
Party Tyme	28
Piña Colada	
Holland House	60
Party Tyme	50
Pink Squirrel	
Holland House	69
Planter's Punch	
Party Tyme	37
Screwdriver	
Holland House	69
Party Tyme	21
Sidecar	
Holland House	17
Sour, Blackberry	
Holland House	50
Sour, Virgin	
Party Tyme	50
Sour, Whiskey	
Canada Dry	11
Holland House	53
Holland House low calorie	9
Party Tyme	29
Party Tyme instant	53
Sip 'n Slim	
Holland House	10

Strawberry Sting	
Holland House	35
Tom Collins	
Holland House	58
Party Tyme	44
Party Tyme instant	58

Cocktails, standard recipe, alcoholic, 1 oz alcohol, unless noted

Bacardi	155
Bloody Mary	140
Brandy Alexander	225
Bourbon Highball (1½ oz bourbon)	
with soda	125
with ginger ale	180
Cuba Libre	224
Daiquiri	135
Gimlet	136
Gin Fizz	172
Grasshopper	235
Irish Coffee	214
Manhattan	177
Martini, Gin or Vodka	115
Mint Julep	209
Old Fashioned	144
Orange Blossom	153
Pink Lady	190
Rob Roy	199

Rum Cola (see Cuba Libre)	224
Screwdriver	168
Side Car	161
Sloe Gin Fizz	155
Stinger	149
Tom Collins	170
Whiskey Sour	142

Wines, 4 oz

Alsatian	
Wilm	88
Altar, red	
Gold Seal	132
Henri Marchant	132
Blackberry	
Manischewitz	180
Bordeaux	
red	
B&G Margaux	83
B&G Prince Noir	81
B&G Saint-Emilion	84
Chanson	108
Cruse	92
Cruse Saint-Emilion	92
Cruse Saint-Julien	92
Cruse Médoc	96
Cruse Château La Garde	108

Cruse Château Olivier	108
white	
B&G Graves	87
Cruse Graves	92
Burgundy	
red	
B&G Beaujolais St. Louis	80
B&G Nuits St. George	93
B&G Pommard	89
Chanson Beaune	108
Chanson Pommard	108
Cruse Beaujolais	96
Cruse Pommard	96
Cruse Gevrey-Chambertin	96
Gallo	67
Gold Seal	86
Henri Marchant	84
Italian Swiss Colony	86
Manischewitz	85
Taylor	99
sparkling	
B&G	92
Chanson	96
Gold Seal	97
Great Western	109
Henri Marchant	97
Lejon	89
Taylor	104
white	
B&G	83

Chanson	108
Gold Seal	85
Henri Marchant	86
Cabernet Sauvignon	
Inglenook	77
Martini	120
Capella	
Italian Swiss Colony	85
Catawba	
pink	
Gold Seal	132
Great Western	148
Henri Marchant	132
Manischewitz	129
Taylor	130
red	
Gold Seal	128
Henri Marchant	132
white	
Gold Seal	132
Henri Marchant	132
Chablis	
Gold Seal	88
Great Western	92
Henri Marchant	90
Inglenook	76
Italian Swiss Colony	89
Taylor	98
Champagne	
Bollinger	114

- *Great Western* — 121
- *Taylor* — 120

Concord
- *Gold Seal* — 132
- *Henri Marchant* — 132
- *Manischewitz*
  - red — 160
  - white — 130
  - medium dry — 120
  - dry — 85
- *Mogen David* — 160

Kosher
- *Manischewitz*
  - sweet — 170
  - medium — 112
  - dry — 91

Labrusca
- *Gold Seal* — 130
- *Henri Marchant* — 132

Lake Country
- *Taylor* — 106

Liebfraumilch
- *Anheuser & Fehrs* — 80
- *Dienhard* — 95

Malaga
- *Manischewitz* — 180

Moselle
- *Dienhard* — 95
- *Julius Kayser* — 77

Great Western	96
Pinot Chardonnay	
Gold Seal	85
Henri Marchant	85
Louis Martini	120
Pinot Noir	
Inglenook	77
Louis Martini	120
Pouilly-Fumé	
B&G	80
Rhine	
Gold Seal	91
Dienhard	80
Gallo	67
Gallo Rhine Garten	78
Great Western	97
Henri Marchant	92
Julius Kayser	74
Inglenook	100
Italian Swiss Colony	86
Louis Martini	120
Taylor	92
Rhineskeller	
Italian Swiss Colony	88
Rice Wine	
Chinese	152
Japanese	286
Rhone	
Chanson	112

B&G	93
Riesling	
Dienhard	96
Gold Seal	92
Henri Marchant	92
Inglenook	82
Louis Martini	120
Rosé	
Cruse	96
Gold Seal	99
Henri Marchant	96
Italian Swiss Colony	86
Taylor	92
Sake	151
Sancerre	
B&G	80
Sauterne	
Gallo	67
Gallo Haut	83
Gold Seal	97
Gold Seal Haut	109
Great Western	105
Henri Marchant	109
Italian Swiss Colony	77
Louis Martini	120
Mogen David cream	59
Mogen David dry	39
Taylor	105
Soave	
Antinori	110

Thunderbird	
Gallo	139
Valpolicella	
Antinori	109
Zinfandel	
Inglenook	76
Italian Swiss Colony	80
Louis Martini	120

Aperitif and Dessert Wines, 4 oz

Asti Spumante	
Gancia	168
Aquavit	
Leroux	300
Campari	66
Dubonnet Blonde	151
Dubonnet Red	190
Madeira	
Gold Seal	144
Henri Marchant	144
Leacock	160
Sandeman	168
Muscatel	
Gallo	144
Gold Seal	210
Pernod	
Julius Wyle	315

Port	
Gallo	146
Gold Seal	185
Great Western	178
Italian Swiss Colony	170
Louis Martini	215
Robertson	180
Sandeman	184
Taylor	195
Sherry	
Gallo	104
Gold Seal	185
Great Western	156
Taylor	200
Dry Sack	160
Sherry, cream	
Gallo	150
Gold Seal	205
Great Western	180
Louis Martini	175
Taylor	178
Sherry, dry	
Gallo	110
Gold Seal	162
Great Western	140
Italian Swiss Colony	132
Louis Martini	180
Sandeman	145
Taylor	152

Vermouth, dry

C&P	148
Gallo	100
Gancia	168
Great Western	113
Lejon	129
Noilly Pratt	136
Taylor	136

Vermouth, sweet

C&P	156
Gallo	150
Gancia	185
Great Western	172
Lejon	174
Noilly Pratt	172
Taylor	175

Cordials and Liqueurs, 1 oz

Amaretto	80
Anise	82
Anisette	
Bols	111
DuBouchett	85
DeKuyper	95
Garnier	82
Mr. Boston	90
Mr. Boston Connoisseur	64

Apricot	
Bols	96
Dolfi	100
DuBouchett	65
B & B	94
Benai	110
Benedictine	110
Blackberry	
Bols	90
Dolfi	89
DuBouchett	68
Brandy, flavored	
Bols	100
DuBouchett	87
Garnier	6
Leroux	90
Mr. Boston	100
Mr. Boston Connoisseur	75
Cherry liqueur	
Bols	96
DeKuyper	75
Dolfi	87
DuBouchett	72
Hiram Walker	82
Leroux	82
Chocolate	
Vandermint	90
Claristine	
Leroux	114

Coffee

Tia Maria	92
Pasha	100

Crème de almond

DuBouchett	100

Crème de apricot

Mr. Boston	90
Mr. Boston Connoisseur	65

Crème de banana

Garnier	90
Mr. Boston	90
Mr. Boston Connoisseur	65

Crème de cacao

Bols	100
Dolfi	100
DuBouchett	100
Garnier	100
Hiram Walker	100
Mr. Boston	90
Mr. Boston Connoisseur	65

Crème de cassis

Leroux	87
Mr. Boston	90
Crème de menthe	100
Crème de noisette	90

Crème de noyaux

Bols	115
Mr. Boston	99

Crème de peach

Mr. Boston Connoisseur	65

Curaçao	100
Drambuie	110
Grenadine	81
Kirsch	80
Kümmel	
DuBouchett	
48 proof	65
70 proof	83
Garnier	75
Hiram Walker	71
Leroux	75
Mr. Boston	78
Lochon Ora	
Leroux	89
Peach Liqueur	
Bols	96
DeKuyper	82
Dolfi	103
DuBouchett	67
Hiram Walker	81
Leroux	85
Raspberry Liqueur	
Dolfi	80
DuBouchett	56
Rock & Rye	
DuBouchett	
60 proof	78
70 proof	86
Garnier	83
Mr. Boston	90

Mr. Boston Connoisseur	65
Schnapps, peppermint	
DuBouchett	85
Garnier	83
Hiram Walker	78
Leroux	87
Mr. Boston	77
Sloe Gin	
Bols	85
DeKuyper	70
Dolfi	114
DuBouchett	70
Garnier	83
Mr. Boston	67
Triple Sec	
Bols	104
Dolfi	107
DuBouchett	61
Garnier	83
Hiram Walker	105
Leroux	104
Mr. Boston	100

BEER, ALE, MALT LIQUOR, 12 oz

Andeker	160
Black Horse Ale	162
Brauhaus	150

Buckeye	144
Budweiser	156
Budweiser Malt Liquor	160
Busch Bavarian	155
Carling Black Label	160
Carlsberg Light	159
Carlsberg Dark	240
Champale Malt Liquor	157
Country Club Malt Liquor	163
Coors	138
Eastside Lager	145
Falstaff	150
Gablinger's	99
Goebel	145
Grand Union	150
Grenzquell	150
Hamms	138
Heidelberg	133
Heidelberg Light	129
Heileman's	158
Kingsbury	146
Knickerbocker	160
Meister Brau	144
Meister Brau Draft	144
Meister Brau Lite	96
Michelob	160
Michelob Light	134
Miller	150
Miller Lite	96
Natural Light	110

Old Dutch	150
Old Milwaukee	144
Old Ranger	150
Pabst Blue Ribbon	150
Pabst Light	100
Pabst Extra Light	70
Pearl	145
Pilser's	152
Red Cap Ale	159
Rheingold	160
Schaefer	158
Schlitz	148
Schlitz Light	96
Schmidt's	142
Stag	151
Stroh Bohemian	136
Stroh Bock	155
Stroh Light	115
Tuborg USA	140
Tudor	150

Near Beer, 12 oz

Goetz Pale	78
Kingsbury	45

1

Nonalcoholic Beer, 12 oz

Maltcrest	70
Metbrew	70
Zing	65

SOFT DRINKS, 8 oz

Note: Virtually all sodas that are called *low calorie*, *sugar free*, or *dietetic* contain 2 calories or less.

Aspen	105
Birch Beer	
Canada Dry	110
Pennsylvania Dutch	109
Yukon Club	116
Bitter lemon	
Canada Dry	104
Schweppes	128
Bitter orange	
Schweppes	124
Bubble Up	97
Cactus Cooler	120
Cherry	
Cott	123
Crush	121

Fanta	117
Mission	122
Club soda, all brands	0
Coconut	
Yoo-Hoo	117
Coffee	
Hoffman	88
Cola	
Canada Dry	110
Coca-Cola	96
Pepsi-Cola	104
Royal Crown	109
Pepsi Light	47
Shasta	90
Cream	
Canada Dry	127
Fanta	130
Shasta	90
Schweppes	115
Dr. Brown's Cel-Ray Tonic	89
Dr. Nehi	98
Dr. Pepper	98
Fruit punch	
Shasta	110
Fruit mix	
Wyler's	88
Ginger Ale	
Canada Dry	85
Fanta	85
Nehi	91

Schweppes	88
Ginger Beer	
Schweppes	96
Grape	
Canada Dry	130
Crush	120
Fanta	114
Nehi	116
Patio	128
Schweppes	129
Shasta	114
Grapefruit	
Fanta	115
Shasta	103
Half and Half	110
Hi Spot	100
Kick	118
***Kool Aid*, all flavors**	93
Lemon	
Hi-C	123
Shasta	97
Lemon-Lime	
Shasta	93
Lime	
Canada Dry	130
Mello-Yello	115
Mr. PiBB	93
Mountain Dew	118
Orange	
Canada Dry	130

Crush	120
Fanta	114
Hi-C	101
Nedick's	121
Nehi	124
Patio	128
Schweppes	118
Shasta	114
Sunkist	125
Pineapple	
Canada Dry	110
Purple Passion	
Canada Dry	120
Quinine Water	
Canada Dry	95
Fanta	84
Schweppes	88
Rondo	
Schweppes	100
Root Beer	
A&W	114
Berks County	116
Canada Dry Barrelhead	110
Canada Dry Rooti	110
Dad's	105
Fanta	103
Hires	100
On Tap	105
Patio	110
Royal Crown	113

Schweppes	105
Shasta	100
7-Up	97
Sprite	95
Squirt	91
Strawberry	
Canada Dry	120
Crush	121
Fanta	121
Nehi	116
Shasta	94
Yoo-Hoo	124
Sun-Drop	118
Teem	93
Tahitian Treat	
Canada Dry	130
Tiki	100
Tonic	
Canada Dry	90
Schweppes	88
Shasta	66
Upper 10	101
Vanilla	
Yoo-Hoo	125
Vanilla Cream	
Canada Dry	130
Wild Cherry	
Canada Dry	130
Wink	120

COFFEE AND TEA, 6 oz

Coffee	
regular	2
instant	4
flavored	
General Foods	
Cafe Francais	60
Cafe Vienna	60
Orange Cappuccino	60
Suisse Mocha	60
Postum	10
Tea, bags or loose	1
Tea, bottled or canned	
Lipton	84
sugar free	1
No-Cal	0
Tea, instant	
Lipton lemon-flavored	3
100% Tea	0
Nestea	1
Tender Leaf	1
Tea, mix, iced, lemon-flavored	
Our Own (A&P)	62
Lipton	40
Nestea	15
with sugar	70

Salada	57
Wyler's	56

FRUIT AND VEGETABLE JUICES, 6 oz

Fresh

Grapefruit	70
Lemon or Lime	45
Lemon or Lime, 1 Tbsp	3
Orange	
California	85
Florida	80
Valencia	85
Peach Nectar	90
Tangerine	80

Bottled and Canned

Apple	
Ann Page	90
Heinz	75

Musselman's	80
Mott's	80
Pillsbury	60
Seneca	80
Welch's	90
Apple-Cranberry	
Lincoln	104
Apricot nectar	
Del Monte	100
Heart's Delight	194
Heinz	104
Libby's	110
Seneca	75
Cranberry-Apple	
Cranapple	120
Fig	
Real Fig	135
Fig and Prune	
Fig 'n' Prune	135
Grape	
Heinz	120
Seneca	110
Welch's	120
Grapefruit	
Del Monte	70
Heinz	70
Libby's	75
Ocean Spray	70
Seneca	55
Stokely-Van Camp	60

Welch's	75
Grapefruit-Orange	
Seneca	77
Grenadine syrup, nonalcoholic, 1 oz.	
Garnier	100
Giroux	104
Lemon, 1 Tbsp	
ReaLemon	4
Rose's	5
Lime, 1 Tbsp	
ReaLime	6
Orange	
Del Monte	80
Heinz	75
Libby's	90
Welch's	90
Orange-Grapefruit	
Del Monte	80
Libby's	80
Stokely-Van Camp	70
Peach Nectar	
Del Monte	100
Libby's	90
Heart's Delight	89
Pear Nectar	
Del Monte	110
Libby's	100
Heart's Delight	95
Pineapple	
Del Monte	100

Dole	93
Heinz	95
Seneca	68
Stokely-Van Camp	110
Pineapple-Grapefruit	
Del Monte	90
Pineapple-Orange	
Ann Page	87
Del Monte	90
Hi-C	94
Lincoln	97
Prune	
Ann Page	140
Del Monte	120
Heinz	130
Mott's	140
RealPrune	130
Seneca	130
Sunsweet	124
Welch's	150
Tomato	
Campbell's	35
Del Monte	35
Heinz	38
Hunt's	43
Libby's	39
Sacramento	32
Seneca	27
Stokely-Van Camp	33
Townhouse	35

Welch's 38

Vegetable

Campbell V-8 35

Vegemato 32

Frozen Juice

Grape

Minute Maid 99

Snow Crop 99

Grapefruit

Bird's Eye 68

Minute Maid 75

Snow Crop 75

Lemon

Minute Maid 40

Orange

Bright and Early 90

Minute Maid 90

Snow Crop 120

Stokely-Van Camp 90

Orange-Grapefruit

Bird's Eye 72

Minute Maid 76

Pineapple

Dole 101

Minute Maid 92

Pineapple-orange	
Minute Maid	94
Dole	77
Tangerine	
Minute Maid	86
Snow Crop	85

Dairy-Packed Juice, 8 oz

Grapefruit	
Tropicana	75
Orange	
Borden	96
Kraft	90
Sealtest	96
Tropicana	83
Orange-Grapefruit	
Kraft	90
Orange-Pineapple	
Ann Page	87
Hi-C	94
Kraft	96

FRUIT-FLAVORED DRINKS, ALL TYPES, 6 oz

Apple

Ann Page	90
Hi-C	90

Apple-Grape

Mott's	90
Welch's	92

Apricot-Apple

BC	92

Cherry

Ann Page	90
Hi-C	75

Citrus Cooler

Ann Page	90
Hi-C	90

Cranberry

Ann Page	120
Ocean Spray	105
Seneca	120
Welch's	105

Cranberry-Apple

Ann Page	135
Lincoln	103
Mott's	95
Ocean Spray	135

Cranberry-Apricot	
Ocean Spray	105
Cranberry-Grape	
Ocean Spray	105
Welch's	120
Cranberry-Orange	
Knox	59
Cranberry-Prune	
Ocean Spray	120
Grape	
Ann Page	90
Hi-C	90
Welch's	90
Grape-Apple	
BC	107
Grapefruit	
Ann Page	80
Sealtest	90
Tropicana	70
Lemon	
Sealtest	90
Lemonade	
Bird's Eye	74
Borden	78
Country Time	67
Hi-C	75
Minute Maid	75
ReaLemon	76
Sealtest	80
Snow Crop	75

Stokely-Van Camp	80
Wyler's	67
Lemon-Limeade	
Minute Maid	75
Snow Crop	75
Limeade	
Bird's Eye	75
Minute Maid	75
Snow Crop	75
Orange	
A&P	80
Ann Page	90
Bird's Eye	105
Borden	85
Hi-C	125
Minute Maid	125
Start	120
Stokely-Van Camp	114
Tang	120
Tropicana	93
Welch's	135
Orange-Pineapple	
Ann Page	120
BC	120
Start	120
Peach	
Hi-C	120
Pineapple-Grapefruit	
Dole	120

Punch

Ann Page	120
Hawaiian Punch	120
Hi-C	130
Mott's	120
Stokely-Van Camp	114
Tropicana	93
Welch's	130
Wyler's	85
Raspberry	
Wyler's	85
Strawberry	
Hi-C	120
Wyler's	85
Tangerine	
Hi-C	120
Wild Berry	
Ann Page	120
Hi-C	115

CHAPTER 2

Dairy

BUTTER AND MARGARINE

Butter	
½ cup (¼ lb)	815
1 Tbsp	100
Butter, whipped	
½ cup	540
1 Tbsp	65
Margarine, 1 Tbsp	
Imitation	
Mazola	50
Parkay	50
Weight Watchers	50

Regular and Soft, all brands	100
Diet, all brands	50
Spread	
Blue Bonnet	80
Fleishmann	80
Parkay	70
Whipped, all brands	70

CHEESE, 1 oz unless noted

American	
Borden	104
Kraft	90
Blue	
Borden	105
Casino	100
Kraft	99
Brie	
Dorman	100
Kraft	100
Camembert	
Borden	85
Kraft	85
Caraway	
Kraft	111
Cheddar	
Borden	113
Kraft	113

Colby	
Borden	111
Kraft	111
Cottage, 1 cup	
creamed	
Borden	240
Breakstone	230
Breakstone low-fat	180
Foremost	212
Friendship	360
Kraft	214
Lucerne	240
Meadow Gold	134
Sealtest	114
partly creamed	
Meadow Gold	204
Sealtest	176
uncreamed, potstyle	
Borden	196
Breakstone	170
Kraft	206
Sealtest	180
low fat	
Borden	180
Breakstone	180
Friendship	200
Lucerne	200
Viva	200
Weight Watchers	180

Cream cheese	
Borden	96
Kraft Philadelphia Brand	98
Edam	
Dorman	105
House of Gold	105
Farmer's	
Breakstone	30
Dutch Garden	100
Friendship	38
Wispride	100
Fondue	
Swiss Knight	60
Fontina	
Kraft	114
Frankenmuth	
Kraft	113
Gjetost	
Kraft	135
Gorgonzola	
Kraft	112
Gouda	
Borden	86
Kraft	108
Gruyère	
Borden	101
Kraft	108
Swiss Knight	101
Leyden	
Kraft	80

Liederkranz	
Borden	86
Limburger	
Borden	97
Dorman	100
Kraft	98
Mountain Valley	100
Monterey Jack	
Borden	103
Casino	100
Kraft	103
Mozzarella	
Borden	79
Kraft	79
Dorman	85
Muenster	
Borden	85
Dorman	90
Kraft	100
Neufchâtel	
Borden	73
Kraft	69
Nuworld	
Kraft	104
Parmesan, grated, 1 Tbsp	
Buitoni	23
Kraft	27
La Rosa	33
Lucerne	25

Parmesan & Romano, grated, 1 Tbsp	
Borden	30
Kraft	30
Pimiento	
Borden	104
Kraft	104
Port Salut	
Dorman	100
Kraft	100
Premost	
Kraft	134
Provolone	
Borden	93
Kraft	99
Ricotta	
Borden	42
Kraft	99
Romano, grated, 1 Tbsp	
Buitoni	21
Kraft	26
Roquefort	
Borden	107
Kraft	105
Sap Sago	
Kraft	76
Sardo Romano	
Kraft	110
Scamorze	
Kraft	100

Swiss
Borden 104
Dorman 90
Kraft 104
Sage
Kraft 113
Tilsit
Dorman 95

Cheese Food

American
Borden 92
Kraft 77
Blue
Borden 82
Borden Vera Blue 91
Wispride 100
Cheddar
Wispride 100
Jalapeno pepper
Kraft 93
Munst-ett
Kraft 101
Pimiento
Borden 91
Pauley Swiss 90
Velveeta 90
Pizza
Kraft 80

Sharp	
Kraft	93
Swiss	
Borden	91
Kraft	91

Cheese Spread

American	
Borden	85
Kraft	77
Kraft Old English	97
American with Bacon	
Borden	80
Kraft	92
Blue	
Borden	82
Roka	80
Wispride	92
Cheddar	
Snack Mate	85
Wispride	97
Garlic	
Borden	82
Kraft	86
Limburger	
Borden	82

Mohawk Valley	70
Moose	70
Pimiento	
Cheez Whiz	76
Kraft	77
Snack Mate	90
Smoked	
Borden	80
Velveeta	80

CREAM, 1 Tbsp

half and half	
Borden	19
Meadow Gold	27
Sealtest	20
light	
Borden	25
Foremost	30
Sealtest	35
medium	
Borden	41
Sealtest	42
heavy (whipping)	
Borden	52

Foremost	52
Lucerne	10
Sealtest	52

Sour Cream, 1 Tbsp

Borden	29
***Borden* half and half**	29
***Borden* imitation**	25
Foremost	30
Sealtest	29

Non-Dairy Creamers, 1 Tsp

coffee creamers	
Carnation Coffee-Mate	11
Meadow Gold	9
Pet Cremora	11
whipped toppings	
Reddi-Whip	7
Sta-Whip	8

EGGS

Chicken	
raw, boiled, or poached	
medium	72
large	82
extra large	94
raw, white only	
medium	15
large	18
extra large	20
1 cup	125
raw, yolk only	
medium	53
large	60
extra large	68
fried	
medium	85
large	97
extra large	113
scrambled or omelet	
medium	99
large	110
extra large	127
Duck, raw	130
Goose, raw	266
Turkey, raw	135

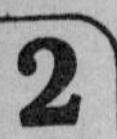

Egg Mixes, Commercial

Imitation

Morningstar Farms Scramblers, ½ cup	130
Tillie Lewis Eggstra, 1 pkt	101
Fleishmann Egg Beaters, ½ cup	81
Omelets, 1 pkt	
Plain	
Durkee	604
Durkee dry mix	112
with bacon	
Durkee	620
Durkee dry mix	125
with cheese	
Durkee	617
Durkee dry mix	127
McCormick	130
Schilling	128
Western	
Durkee	604
Durkee dry mix	112
McCormick	115
Schilling	115
Scrambled	
Durkee	124
with bacon	
Durkee	180
with sausage and potatoes	
Swanson	452

MILK, 8 oz

Buttermilk	
Borden	
.1% fat	88
.5% fat	90
1% fat	107
1.5% fat	110
2% fat	122
3% fat	158
Friendship 1.4% fat	120
Golden Nugget .8%	92
Light 'n Lively .8% fat	95
Lucerne 1.5% fat	120
Sealtest 2% fat	114
Skim	
Borden .1% fat	81
Lucerne	
0% fat	90
1% fat	110
2% fat	130
Meadow Gold	
.5% fat	87
2% fat	130
Sealtest .1% fat	79
Skim Fortified	
Borden	81
Borden Lite Line	117
Borden Hi Protein	132

Gail Borden	81
Light 'n Lively	114
Sealtest	137
Whole	
Borden	160
Foremost	154
Lucerne	160
Meadow Gold	166
Sealtest	150
Whole Fortified	
Gail Borden	159
Sealtest Multivitamin	151

Milk Beverages, 8 oz unless noted

Cherry-vanilla	
Borden	291
Chocolate	
Borden	210
Meadow Gold	190
Sealtest	175
Chocolate fudge	
Borden	284
Chocolate mixes	
Carnation Instant, 1 pkt	130
Carnation Slender, 1 pkt	110
Nestle's Quik	215

Ovaltine, 1 oz 105
Pillsbury, 1 pkt 295
Safeway, 2 tsp 215
Sealtest 195
Chocolate malt mix
Carnation Instant, 1 pkt 130
Carnation Slender, 1 pkt 110
Eggnog, dairy packed
Borden
4.7% fat 260
6% fat 302
8% fat 375
Carnation, 1 pkt 130
Meadow Gold 327
Sealtest 324
Malt
Borden 80
Carnation 90
Ovaltine 100
Mocha
Borden 291
Strawberry
Borden 287
Carnation, 1 pkt 130
Pillsbury, 1 pkt 290
Vanilla
Borden 291
Carnation, 1 pkt 130

YOGURT, 8 oz

Plain	
Borden Lite-Line	140
Borden Swiss Style	167
Breakstone	144
Dannon	150
Light 'n Lively	140
Lucerne	160
Pet	157
Viva	180
Flavored, all flavors	
Borden	270
Breyer's	270
Dannon	210
Light 'n Lively	240
Meadow Gold	270
Viva	250
Frozen	
Danny	
In-A-Cup, 8 oz.	180
On-A-Stick, uncoated	65

CHAPTER 3

Breads, Crackers, Flour

BREAD, 1 slice, approximately 1 oz unless noted

Bran	
Brownberry	75
Corn & Molasses	
Pepperidge Farm	71
Cinnamon Raisin	
Thomas	60
Cracked Wheat	
Pepperidge Farm	66

Tasty Bake	70
Date Nut	
Thomas	100
French	
Pepperidge Farm	79
Wonder	75
Garlic	
Stouffer	80
Gluten	
Thomas	32
Hollywood	70
Honey Bran	
Pepperidge Farm	58
Honey Wheatberry	
Arnold	90
Pepperidge Farm	60
Italian	
Pepperidge Farm	81
Naturel	
Arnold	65
Nut	
Brownberry	85
Oatmeal	
Brownberry	82
Pepperidge Farm	66
Profile	52
Protein	
Thomas	45
Pumpernickel	
Arnold	75

Pepperidge Farm	79
Raisin	
Plain	
Arnold	75
Thomas	66
with cinnamon	
Brownberry	85
Pepperidge Farm	75
Thomas	65
with nuts	
Brownberry	95
Rice Cakes	
Spiral	36
Rye	
Arnold	50
Jewish	75
soft	75
Brownberry	65
Pepperidge Farm	82
Tasty Bake	91
Wonder	75
Sourdough	
Di Carlo	71
Wheat	
Arnold	
Granary	71
Branola	90
Brick Oven	60
Melba Thin	40
Brownberry	85

Item	Calories
Buckwheat	75
Colonial	72
Home Pride	75
Pepperidge Farm	70
Pepperidge Farm Very Thin	40
Thomas	50
Wonder	75
Wheat Germ	
Pepperidge Farm	69
White	
Arnold	
Brick Oven, .8 oz slice	65
Brick Oven, 1.1 oz slice	85
Country	95
Hearthstone Country	70
Melba Thin	40
Brownberry Sandwich	75
Brownberry Thin	70
Butternut	75
Colonial	75
Daffodil Farm	58
Fresh Horizons	50
Hart	75
Heartstone	85
Home Pride	75
Homestyle	75
Manor	75
Pepperidge Farm	75
Pepperidge Farm Sandwich	72
Sweetheart	75

Tasty Bake	72
Thomas	64
Weight Watchers	35
Wonder	75
Whole Wheat	
Pepperidge Farm	61
Thomas	65

Bread, Canned, ½ inch slice

Banana Nut	
Dromedary	71
Brown	
B&M	52
Chocolate Nut	
Cross & Blackwell	65
Dromedary	87
Date Nut	
Dromedary	75
Fruit and Nut	
Cross & Blackwell	77
Orange Nut	
Cross & Blackwell	76
Dromedary	78
Spice Nut	
Cross & Blackwell	65

Bread Mixes

White, ¼ loaf	
Pillsbury	460
Cornbread, 1 pkg	
Pillsbury	320
Aunt Jemima	330

BISCUITS, MUFFINS AND ROLLS

Biscuits, Baking Powder, 1 biscuit

1869 Brand	105
prebaked	100
Pillsbury	70
Tenderflake	60

Biscuits, refrigerated, 1 biscuit

Plain	
Ballard	50
Borden	59
Hungry Jack	95
Flaky	90

Pillsbury	55
Flaky Baking Powder	67
Tenderflake	
Baking Powder	60
Buttermilk	
Hungry Jack	
Extra Rich	65
Flaky	80
Fluffy	100
Pillsbury	50
Big Country	95
Extra Light	55
Tenderflake	55
Corn Bread	
Pillsbury	95

Muffins, frozen, 1 muffin

Blueberry	
Thomas	110
Howard Johnson	121
Morton	120
Rounds	110
Pepperidge Farm	130
Corn	
Howard Johnson	118
Morton	
regular	130

Rounds	125
Pepperidge Farm	140
Thomas	120
English	
Thomas	130
Orange	
Howard Johnson	115
Raisin Bran	
Pepperidge Farm	130

Muffins, Mix, 1 muffin

Apple Cinnamon	
Betty Crocker	160
Banana Nut	
Betty Crocker	185
Blueberry	
Betty Crocker	120
Corn	
Betty Crocker	160
Orange	
Betty Crocker	155
Pineapple	
Betty Crocker	125

Muffins, packaged

Bran	
Thomas	118
Cinnamon Raisin	
Pepperidge Farm	140
Corn	
Thomas	180
Toast-r-Cakes	120
English	
Di Carlo	145
Hostess	145
Thomas	140
Wonder	144
Honey Butter	
Arnold Orowheat	150
Onion	
Thomas	130
Raisin	
Wonder	155
Sourdough	
Wonder	130
Wheat	
Home Pride	140

Muffins, refrigerated, 1 muffin

Apple Cinnamon	
Pillsbury	155
Corn	
Pillsbury	130

Rolls, 1 roll

Hard Rolls	
Pepperidge Farm	120
French, 3 oz	264
French, 5 oz	395
Hearth	64
Sesame Crisp	76
Wonder	82
Sandwich and Hamburger Rolls	
Arnold	
Dutch Egg Buns	130
Francisco	180
Soft	110
Hamburger	110
Hot Dog	110
Colonial	160
Pepperidge Farm	120
Wonder	160
Soft Rolls	
Arnold	

Deli-Twist	110
Finger, 24's and 12's	55
Francisco	100
Refrigerator	95
Ballard	95
Borden	
Gem Flake	70
Onion	95
Colonial	80
Home Pride	90
Pepperidge Farm	
Butter Crescent	130
Dinner	65
Finger	60
Golden Twist	120
Old Fashioned	37
Parkerhouse	60
Party	35
Pillsbury	
Butterflake	110
Crescent	95
Hot Roll Mix	95
Wonder	
Buttermilk	85
Pan	105
Sweet Rolls, refrigerated	
Caramel	
Pillsbury	160
Cinnamon	
Ballard	100

Hungry Jack	145
Pillsbury	114
Orange	
Pillsbury	130
Scones	
Hostess	188

CRACKERS, 1 piece

Bacon Flavored	
Keebler	15
Nabisco Bacon Thins	11
Barbecue	
Chit Chat	14
Sunshine	17
Butter	
Hi-Ho	17
Keebler	
Butter Thins	17
Club	15
Townhouse	19
Nabisco	15
Ritz	17
Tam-Tams	13
Butter-cheese	
Ritz	18

Caraway	
Caraway Crazy	15
Cheese	
Cheese-Nips	5
Cheese Tid-Bits	4
Cheez-It	6
Che-Zo	5
Keebler	11
Pepperidge Farm	12
Cheese-peanut Butter	
Keebler	14
Chicken	
Chicken In a Biskit	10
Club	
Keebler	15
Flings Curls	
Nabisco	10
Gold Fish	
Pepperidge Farm, 1 oz	140
Ham	
Nabisco	12
Hi-Ho	
Sunshine	18
Kavli Flatbread	35
Matzos	
Goodman's Square	110
Goodman's Tea	75
Horowitz-Margareten	130
Manischewitz	
Egg	132

Egg 'N Onion	113
Regular	110
Tam Tams	14
Tasteas	115
Thin Tea	110
Whole Wheat	122
Onion	
Keebler	15
Manischewitz	13
Nabisco	13
French Onion	12
Pepperidge Farm	12
Potato	
Chippers	14
Potato Piffles	17
Ritz	
Nabisco	17
Rye	
Keebler Rye Toast	18
Peek Frean	30
Ry Krisp	24
Saltines	
Jacob's	
Biscuits for Cheese	35
English Cream	110
Keebler	
Salt-Free	15
Saltines	14
Sea Toast	60
Whole Wheat Sea Toast	58

Nabisco	
Premium	12
Royal Lunch	54
Uneeda	22
Sunshine	11
Sesame	
Keebler	16
Meal Mates	22
Sesame Sillys	15
Sunshine	24
Shapies	10
Sip'N Chips	10
Sociables	
Nabisco	10
Toasts	
Dutch Rusk	60
Holland Rusk	39
Keebler	15
Old London	11
Pepperidge Farm	11
Sunshine All-Rye	21
Soda and water crackers	
Huntley & Palmer	35
Jacob's Golden Puffs	34
Keebler Milk Lunch	27
Waldorf	18
Zesta	14
Tomato-onion	
Sunshine	15

Town House	
Keebler	**15**
Triangle Thins	
Nabisco	**8**
Twigs	
Nabisco	**14**
Waffle crackers	**22**
Waverly wafers	
Nabisco	**18**
Wheat	
Nabisco	
Wheat Toast	**15**
Wheat Thins	**9**
Zwieback	
Nabisco	**31**

OTHER BREAD PRODUCTS

Breadcrumbs, 1 cup	**450**
Contadina	**450**
4C plain	**410**
4C seasoned	**400**

Breadsticks, 1 piece

onion	
Stella D'Oro	35
plain	
Stella D'Oro	40
sesame	
Stella D'Oro	38
dietetic	
Stella D'Oro	43

Croutons, ½ cup unless noted

bacon	
Bel Air	80
Brownberry	90
cheese and garlic	
Bel Air	100
garlic	
Bel Air	80
Italian cheese	
Bel Air	100
plain	
Bel Air	60
seasoned	
Bel Air	90
Brownberry	90

Stuffing, mixes, 1 pkg

Pepperidge Farm	110
Stove Top	170
Uncle Ben's	120

FLOURS, 1 cup

Buckwheat	
dark	325
light	340
Cake	370
Carob	250
Corn	485
Corn Starch, 1 Tbsp	35
Lima Bean	430
Peanut	225
Rye	
light	315
medium	310
dark	420
Soybean, defatted	325
full fat	300
low fat	310
Tortilla	
corn	410

wheat	450
Wheat, all purpose	485
bread	500
cake	430
gluten	530
self-rising	440
whole wheat	400
White	400
Unbleached	400

Meal, 1 cup

Almond	696
Corn	433
Cracker	450
Graham cracker	465
Matzo	444

CHAPTER 4

Cereal, Pancakes, Waffles and French Toast

CEREAL, ready to eat, 1 cup

bran	
All-Bran, *Kellogg's*	190
40% Bran Flakes, *Kellogg's*	140
100% Bran Flakes, *Nabisco*	150
40% Bran Flakes, *Post*	125
Bran Chex, *Ralston Purina*	165
Bran & Prune Flakes, *Post*	120
Bran & Raisin Flakes, *General Mills*	125
Raisin Bran, *Kellogg's*	200
Raisin Bran, *Ralston Purina*	200
Raisin Bran, *Safeway*	200

Raisin Bran with Sugar Coating, *Post*	178
Bran-Buds with wheat germ, *Kellogg's*	200
corn	
Country Corn Flakes, *General Mills*	80
Kix, *General Mills*	75
Corn Flakes, *Kellogg's*	110
Toasties Corn Flakes, *Post*	110
Corn Chex, *Ralston Purina*	110
Corn Flakes, *Ralston Purina*	110
Corn Flakes, *Safeway*	110
Corn Flakes & Blueberries, *Post*	110
Corn Flakes & Strawberries, *Post*	110
Sugar Frosted Flakes, *Kellogg's*	144
Sugar Pops, *Kellogg's*	105
Honeycomb Corn, *Post*	85
Sugar Sparkled Flakes, *Post*	149
Cocoa Puffs, *General Mills*	110
Trix, *General Mills*	111
corn and oats	
Sugar Sparkled Twinkies, *General Mills*	112
Cap'n Crunch, *Quaker*	163
Crisp, *Quaker*	105
oats	
Cheerios, *General Mills*	110
OK's, *Kellogg's*	83
Alpha-Bits, *Post*	110
Crispy Critters, *Post*	110
Fortified Oat Flakes, *Post*	165
Life, *Quaker*	160
Lucky Charms, *General Mills*	110

Frosty O's, *General Mills*	110
Sugar Jets, *General Mills*	111
Stars, *Kellogg's*	112
Fruit Loops, *Kellogg's*	112
rice	
Rice Krispies, *Kellogg's*	105
Puffed Rice, *Quaker*	45
Crispy Rice, *Ralston Purina*	110
Rice Chex, *Ralston*	110
Crispy Rice, *Safeway*	110
Puffa Puffa Rice, *Kellogg's*	120
Rice Honeys, *Nabisco*	150
Rice Krinkles, *Post*	127
Cocoa Crispies, *Kellogg's*	113
wheat	
Buc Wheats, *General Mills*	146
Total, *General Mills*	110
Wheat Stax, *General Mills*	81
Wheaties, *General Mills*	108
Crumbles, *Kellogg's*	140
Pep, *Kellogg's*	106
Shredded Wheat, *Kellogg's* 1 biscuit	63
Shredded Wheat, *Nabisco* 1 biscuit	92
Grape Nuts Flakes, *Post*	150
Puffed Wheat, *Quaker*	38
Shredded Wheat, *Quaker* 1 biscuit	68
Wheat Chex, *Ralston Purina*	165
Sugar Crisp, *Kellogg's*	147
Sugar Smacks, *Kellogg's*	110
Wheat Honeys, *Nabisco*	153

mixed grains	
Concentrate, *Kellogg's*	310
Product 19, *Kellogg's*	106
Special K, *Kellogg's*	70
Apple Jacks, *Kellogg's*	112
Team Flakes, *Nabisco*	83
Grape Nuts, *Post*	400
Quake, *Quaker*	118

Cereal, cooked, 1 cup

barley	
Quaker	172
corn meal mush	
Quaker	128
farina	
Cream of Wheat	
Instant	133
Mix'N Eat	140
Quick	133
Regular	133
H-O	168
Pillsbury	120
Quaker	100
grits	
Quaker	
Instant	79

Instant with cheese flavor, 1 pkt	105
Instant with imitation bacon, 1 pkt	100
Instant with imitation ham, 1 pkt	100
3-Minute Brand, ¼ cup	150
oats	
H-O	150
Quaker	160
oatmeal	
Quaker	143
rice	
Cream of Rice	145
rye	
Con Agra	360
whole wheat	
Quaker Pettilohns	145

PANCAKES, FRENCH TOAST, WAFFLES AND OTHER BREAKFASTS, 1 piece unless noted

Breakfast Bars, frozen	
Carnation	210
General Mills	190

Crepes, mix, 6″ crepe	
Aunt Jemima	55
French Toast, frozen	
Aunt Jemima	85
with cinnamon	100
Downyflake	135
Swanson, with sausage, 1 pkg	335
French Toast, mix	
McCormick	119
Fritters, frozen	
Mrs. Paul's	120
Pancakes, frozen	
Downyflake	75
Swanson, with sausage, 1 pkg	500
Pancakes, frozen batter	
Aunt Jemima	70
Pancakes, mix, 4″ pancake	
Aunt Jemima	
Easy Pour	60
buckwheat	80
buttermilk	70
Betty Crocker	70
Hungry Jack	75
blueberry	112
buttermilk	80
Extra Lights	60
Pancake-Waffle, mix	
Aunt Jemima	70
buttermilk	100
whole wheat	80

Log Cabin	60
buttermilk	75
Waffle, mix	
Aunt Jemima	100
Downyflake	60
Jumbo	89

CHAPTER 5

Beans, Pasta and Rice

BARLEY, 1 cup

pearled, light	698
pearled, Pot or Scotch	696

BEANS DRIED, 1 cup unless noted

Broadbeans, raw, immature seeds, 8 oz	238
Broadbeans, raw, mature seeds, 8 oz	768

Black, dry, uncooked, 8 oz	**768**
Chick peas	
8 oz	**817**
1 cup	**720**
Great Northern	**212**
Lima, immature seeds	**190**
Lima, mature seeds, dried	**262**
Mung, dried	**714**
Pea or Navy, dried	**224**
Pinto (red Mexican), uncooked	**663**
Red Kidney	**220**
White, dried	**224**

Baked Beans, ½ cup

B & M	**180**
Campbell	**148**
barbecue	**171**
with franks	**181**
with pork	**147**
Heinz	**140**
Campside	**180**
with franks	**184**
with pork	**150**
Howard Johnson's	**163**
Morton House	**160**

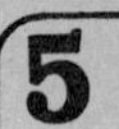

PASTA, 1 cup unless noted

Dry

egg noodles	
Goodman's	175
La Rosa	190
La Rosa spinach	200
Pennsylvania Dutch	200
Prince	190
Ronzoni	200
macaroni	
Goodman's	170
La Rosa	180
Prince	170
Ronzoni	175
spaghetti	
Buitoni	175
Goodman's	160
La Rosa	165
Prince	160
Ronzoni	165

5

Macaroni, canned, bagged, frozen and mixes

with beef	
Banquet	260
Chef Boy-Ar-Dee	235
Franco-American	220
Green Giant Boil-in-Bag, 1 pkg	240
Morton	260
Stouffer's, 1 pkg	380
with beef and cheese	
Banquet	300
Green Giant Boil-in-Bag, 1 pkg	330
Hormel, 7½ oz can	340
Howard Johnson's	330
Morton	215
Mac-A-Roni & Cheddar	290
Pennsylvania Dutch	310
Stouffer's, 1 pkg	520
Swanson	200
with cheese sauce	
Franco-American	225
Heinz	230
MacaroniO's	180
Noodle-Roni	290
Scallop-A-Roni	275
with chili sauce	
Fiesta Mac-A-Roni	270
creole style	
Heinz, 8¾-oz can	169

Noodles, canned, frozen and mixes

Almondine	
Betty Crocker, 1 pkg	960
with beef	
Heinz, 8½ oz can	170
with beef in gravy	
College Inn	238
with beef in tomato sauce	
College Inn	238
with beef	
Hormel, 7½-oz can	240
with beef sauce	
Pennsylvania Dutch	260
Betty Crocker	170
with butter sauce	
Pennsylvania Dutch	300
with cheese	
Noodle-Roni	650
with cheese sauce	
Pennsylvania Dutch	300
with cheese sauce and sour cream	
Noodle-Roni Romanoff	362
with chicken	
Dinty Moore, 7½-oz can	215
with chicken sauce	
Noodle-Roni	250
Pennsylvania Dutch	300
Twist-A-Roni	250

Romanoff	
Betty Crocker, 1 pkg	800
Stouffer's, 1 pkg	500
Stroganoff	
Betty Crocker, 1 pkg	900
Pennsylvania Dutch	630
with tuna	
Stouffer's, 1 pkg	400

Noodles, Italian style, canned, frozen and mixes

Cannelloni, 8 oz	
Weight Watchers	275
Eggplant Parmigiana, 8 oz	
Buitoni	421
Weight Watchers	172
Lasagna, 8 oz unless noted	
Buitoni	250
with meat sauce	340
Chef Boy-Ar-Dee	
canned	241
mix	265
Golden Grain, 1 pkg	720
Green Giant	
Boil-in-Bag, 1 pkg	310
Oven Bake, 1 pkg	300
Hormel	
7½-oz can	270
10-oz can	370

Lean Cuisine, 11 oz	260
Lean Line, 10 oz	270
Roman	274
Stouffer's, 1 pkg	385
Swanson, 1 pkg	540
Weight Watchers	215
Manicotti, 8 oz	
Buitoni	395
with sauce	350
Lean Line	270
Ravioli, 8 oz	
Buitoni	
cheese	575
meat	680
Chef Boy-Ar-Dee	
cheese	263
meat	210
Franco-American, 7½-oz can	220
La Rosa	
cheese	205
meat	218
Roman	
cheese	496
meat	552
Ravioli Parmigiana, 8 oz	
Buitoni	
cheese	301
meat	381

Rotini

Franco-American, 7½-oz can	200
with meatballs	230

Shells

Buitoni, 8 oz	235
Lean Line, 11 oz	270

Spaghetti, all with tomato sauce, 1 cup unless noted

Banquet with meatballs	212
Betty Crocker, 1 pkg	170
Buitoni	
with meatballs	250
with mushrooms	170
Chef Boy-Ar-Dee	
with cheese sauce	180
with meat	260
with meat sauce	250
with meatballs	250
with mushrooms	225
Franco-American	
with cheese sauce	200
with meat	290
with meatballs	260
Spaghetti-Os	
with cheese	200
with meatballs	228
Golden Grain	275
Green Giant, Boil-in-Bag	
with meatballs	280

Heinz	
with cheese sauce	175
with franks	310
with meat sauce	173
Hormel	
with meat	280
with meat sauce	205
Kraft	260
La Rosa with meatballs	230
Lean Cuisine	280
Libby's with meatballs	95
Morton, frozen, 1 pkg	220
Stouffer's, 1 pkg	445
Swanson, 1 pkg	290
Ziti	
Buitoni, 8 oz	270
Lean Line, 10 oz	270
Weight Watchers, 1 pkg	350

RICE, 1 cup unless noted

Plain	
Ann Page, whole pkg	1000
Bird's Eye	260
Carolina	200

Green Giant	230
Minute	300
Rice-A-Roni, whole pkg	780
River	200
Uncle Ben's	200
Uncle Ben's, brown	250
Flavored	
beef	
Uncle Ben's	210
beef and cracked rice	
Betty Crocker	416
beef and vermicelli	
Minute	300
Rice-A-Roni	315
beef and cheese sauce	
Betty Crocker	350
chicken	
Uncle Ben's	210
chicken with crumb topping	
Betty Crocker	365
chicken and vermicelli	
Minute	300
Rice-A-Roni	321
curry	
Uncle Ben's	205
fried Chinese and vermicelli	
Rice-A-Roni	375
ham and vermicelli	
Rice-A-Roni	300

pilaf	
Uncle Ben's	290
Frozen	
Green Giant	160
Medley	220
Pilaf	240
Verdi	140
Spanish, canned	
Heinz	190
La Rosa	155
Libby's	57
Stokely-Van Camp	180

Bulgur (parboiled wheat), 1 cup

Club Wheat, dry	630
Hard Red Winter Wheat, dry	605
canned, unseasoned	225
seasoned	246
White Wheat, dry	555

CHAPTER 6

Soup

CANNED OR FROZEN,
1 cup unless noted

Alphabet	
Golden Grain	55
Alphabet vegetable	
Lipton	68
Asparagus, cream of	
Campbell's	165
Bean	
plain	
Manischewitz	112
Wyler's	95

with bacon
Ann Page 140
Campbell's 174
Town House 155
with hot dogs
Campbell's 168
with smoked pork
Heinz 160
Bean, black
Campbell's 95
Crosse & Blackwell 118
Bean, lima
Manischewitz 93
Beef
plain
Campbell's 105
Lipton 200
with barley
Manischewitz 83
Wyler's 72
with cabbage
Manischewitz 62
with low sodium
Campbell's, 7¼-oz can 170
mushroom
Lipton 45
with noodles
Campbell's 69
Heinz 74
Manischewitz 65

Lipton	67
Souptime, 1 envelope	30
Town House	75
Wyler's	50
with vegetables	
Manischewitz	61
Borscht	
Manischewitz	72
Rokeach	75
Bouillon, 1 cube	
beef	
Herb-Ox	6
Knorr-Swiss	15
Maggi	6
Wyler's	7
chicken	
Herb-Ox	6
Knorr-Swiss	17
Maggi	7
Wyler's	8
onion	
Herb-Ox	10
Wyler's	8
vegetable	
Herb-Ox	6
Wyler's	6
Bouillon, instant, 1 tsp	
beef	
Maggi	6
Wyler's	10

chicken	
Maggi	7
Wyler's	6
Broth	
beef	
Campbell's	26
College Inn	15
Swanson, 6¾-oz can	25
Weight Watchers, 1 pkt	10
chicken	
Campbell's	43
College Inn	32
Richardson & Robbins	17
Swanson, 6¼-oz can	25
chicken with noodles	
College Inn	45
chicken with rice	
College Inn	45
Richardson & Robbins	45
Celery, cream of	
Ann Page	60
Campbell's	160
Heinz	180
Town House	100
Cheddar cheese	
Campbell's	150
Chickarina	
Progresso	100
Chicken	
Lipton	220

Chicken alphabet	
Campbell's	88
Chicken with barley	
Manischewitz	83
Chicken, cream of	
Ann Page	90
Lipton	106
Souptime, 1 pkt	100
Town House	95
Chicken with dumplings	
Campbell's	100
Chicken gumbo	
Campbell's	59
Chicken with kasha	
Manischewitz	41
Chicken with low sodium	
Campbell's, 7½-oz can	170
Chicken noodle	
A & P	67
Ann Page	70
Campbell's	66
Golden Grain	74
Heinz	35
Lipton	54
Manischewitz	46
Souptime, 1 pkt	30
Town House	75
Wyler's	44
Chicken with rice	
Ann Page	50

Campbell's	51
Heinz	58
Lipton	59
Manischewitz	48
Town House	60
Wyler's	49
Chicken with stars	
Ann Page	65
Campbell's	60
Chicken with vegetables	
Ann Page	80
Campbell's	73
Heinz	85
Lipton	70
Manischewitz	55
Town House	85
Wyler's, mix	28
Chili, with beef	
Campbell's	165
Heinz	160
Town House	160
Chowder	
clam, Manhattan	
Campbell's	77
Doxsee	62
Heinz	74
Howard Johnson's	104
Crosse & Blackwell	75
clam, New England	
Campbell's	206

Crosse & Blackwell	124
Doxsee	139
Howard Johnson's	160
Progresso	100
Snow's	148
corn	
Snow's	154
fish	
Snow's	134
Crab	
Crosse & Blackwell	73
Gazpacho	
Crosse & Blackwell	74
Leek, cream of	
Knorr-Swiss	73
Lentil	
La Rosa	137
Manischewitz	166
Progresso	150
Lobster, cream of	
Crosse & Blackwell	113
Meatball Alphabet	
Campbell's	126
Minestrone	
Ann Page	80
Campbell's	88
Golden Grain	66
La Rosa	116

Mushroom	
Plain	
Campbell's	80
Golden Grain	95
Souptime	80
Wyler's	151
with barley	
Manischewitz	72
bisque	
Crosse & Blackwell	127
cream of	
Ann Page	120
Campbell's	217
Heinz	200
Knorr-Swiss	116
Lipton	92
Town House	124
Wyler's	151
Noodle	
Lipton	50
with chicken broth	
Ann Page, 1 pkt	225
Lipton	60
with ground beef	
Campbell's	98
Onion	
Ann Page, 1 pkt	125
Crosse & Blackwell	57
Golden Grain	33

Knorr-Swiss	45
Lipton	35
Souptime, 1 pkt	20
Wyler's	146
Onion with mushroom	
Lipton	35
Oriental style	
Lipton	210
Oyster stew	
Campbell's	
canned	146
frozen	196
Pea	
green	
Campbell's	148
Golden Grain	73
Knorr-Swiss	71
Lipton	136
Souptime low sodium, 1 pkt	70
with ham	
Campbell's	130
low sodium, 7½-oz can	150
split	
Manischewitz	133
split with ham	
Ann Page	180
Campbell's	180
Heinz	150
Town House	154

Pepper pot
Campbell's 105
Petite Marmite
Crosse & Blackwell 41
Potato
Plain
Lipton 100
cream of
Campbell's 190
with leek
Wyler's 155
Schav
Manischewitz 11
Rokeach 12
Scotch broth
Campbell's 90
Senegalese
Crosse & Blackwell 75
Shrimp, cream of
Crosse & Blackwell 113
Campbell's 230
Sirloin burger
Campbell's 177
Steak and potato
Campbell's 160
Stockpot
vegetable
Lipton 220
vegetable-beef
Campbell's 96

Tomato	
Ann Page	80
Campbell's	84
Heinz	87
Lipton	93
Manischewitz	61
Progresso	110
Souptime, 1 pkt	70
Town House	87
Tomato bisque	
Campbell's	126
Tomato	
low sodium	
Campbell's 7¼-oz can	130
with rice	
Ann Page	90
Campbell's	106
Manischewitz	78
with vegetables	
Golden Grain	86
Lipton	69
Tuna Creole	
Crosse & Blackwell	70
Turkey	
Plain	
Campbell's	138
with noodles	
Ann Page	75

Heinz	83
Lipton	74
Town House	83
low sodium	
Campbell's, 7¼-oz can	60
with vegetables	
Ann Page	60
Campbell's	78
Vegetable	
Plain	
Ann Page	70
Campbell's	83
Old Fashioned	74
Lipton	70
Italian	100
Knorr-Swiss	56
Manischewitz	63
Town House	83
Wyler's	81
with beef	
Ann Page	80
Campbell's	81
low sodium, 7¼-oz can	80
Old Fashioned	79
Heinz	66
Lipton	53
Town House	66
cream of	
Souptime, 1 pkt	80

Vegetarian

Campbell's 76

Heinz 83

Vichyssoise

Crosse & Blackwell 140

CHAPTER 7

Meat, Poultry and Seafood

MEAT, FRESH

Retail cuts of meat are frequently weighed with bone first, *then* they are trimmed, cooked and weighed for their yield. So for instance 1 lb. of pork loin chops are weighed raw with bone, but after they are trimmed and cooked, their yield is 5.9 oz.

Beef, choice-grade, retail cuts

Item	Calories
Chuck, arm, roast, or steak; boneless, lean with fat	
raw, 1 lb	1,012
braised, drained	
10.7 oz (yield from 1 lb)	879
4 oz	328
1 cup, chopped	405
1 cup, ground	318
Chuck, arm, roast, or steak, lean only	
braised, drained	
9.1 oz (yield from 1 lb)	498
4 oz	219
1 cup, chopped	270
1 cup, diced	212
Chuck, rib roast or steak, lean with fat	
raw, 1 lb	1,597
braised, drained	
10.7 oz (yield from 1 lb)	1,298
4 oz	484
1 cup, chopped	598
1 cup, ground	470
Chuck, stewing; boneless, lean with fat	
raw, 1 lb	1,166
stewed, drained	
10.7 oz (yield from 1 lb)	994
4 oz	371
1 cup, chopped	458
Chuck, stewing; boneless, lean only	
raw, 1 lb	717

stewed, drained	
10.7 oz (yield from 1 lb)	651
4 oz	243
1 cup, chopped	300
Club steak, 16% bone, lean with fat	
raw, 1 lb	1,443
broiled	
9.8 oz (yield from 1 lb raw)	1,262
4 oz without bone	515
Club steak, 16% bone, lean only	
broiled	
5.7 oz (yield from 1 lb)	393
4 oz without bone	277
Flank steak, boneless, lean only	
raw, 1 lb	653
braised, drained	
10.7 oz (yield from 1 lb)	596
4 oz	222
Ground, lean with 10% fat	
raw, 1 lb	812
broiled, 12 oz (yield from 1 lb)	745
Ground, lean with 21% fat	
raw, 1 lb	1,216
broiled, 11.5 oz (yield from 1 lb)	932
Plate, boneless, lean with fat	
raw, 1 lb	1,216
simmered, drained	
10.7 oz (yield from 1 lb)	1,313
4 oz	490

Plate, boneless, lean only	
simmered, drained	
6.5 oz (yield from 1 lb)	368
4 oz	226
Porterhouse steak, 9% bone, lean with fat	
raw, 1 lb	1,603
broiled	
10.6 oz (yield from 1 lb)	1,400
4 oz without bone	527
Porterhouse steak, 9% bone, lean only	
broiled	
6.1 oz (yield from 1 lb)	385
4 oz without bone	254
Rib roast, boneless, lean with fat	
raw, 1 lb	1,819
roasted	
11.7 oz (yield from 1 lb)	1,456
4 oz	499
1 cup, chopped	616
1 cup, ground	484
Rib roast, boneless, lean only	
roasted	
7.5 oz (yield from 1 lb)	511
4 oz	273
1 cup, chopped	337
1 cup, ground	265
Round steak, boneless, lean with fat	
raw, 1 lb	894
braised or broiled	
11.1 oz (yield from 1 lb)	820

4 oz	296
Round steak, boneless, lean only	
braised or broiled	
9.5 oz (yield from 1 lb)	507
4 oz	296
Rump roast, boneless, lean with fat	
raw, 1 lb	1,374
roasted	
11.7 oz (yield from 1 lb)	1,149
4 oz	394
1 cup, chopped	486
1 cup, ground	382
Rump roast, boneless, lean only	
roasted	
8.8 oz (yield from 1 lb)	516
4 oz	236
1 cup, chopped	291
1 cup, ground	229
Sirloin steak, double bone, 18% bone, lean with fat	
raw, 1 lb	1,240
broiled	
9.6 oz (yield from 1 lb)	1,110
4 oz without bone	463
Sirloin steak, double bone, 18% bone, lean only	
broiled	
6.3 oz (yield from 1 lb)	372
4 oz without bone	272
Sirloin steak, round-bone, 7% bone, lean with fat	
raw, 1 lb	1,316

broiled	
10.9 oz (yield from 1 lb)	1,192
4 oz without bone	439
Sirloin steak, round-bone, 7% bone, lean only	
broiled	
7.2 oz (yield from 1 lb)	420
4 oz without bone	235
T-bone steak, 11% bone, lean with fat	
raw, 1 lb	1,596
broiled	
10.4 oz (yield from 1 lb)	1,395
4 oz without bone	537
T-bone steak, 11% bone, lean only	
broiled	
5.8 oz (yield from 1 lb)	368
4 oz without bone	253

Beef, prepared and specialty cuts

Beef, corned	
raw, 1 lb	1,596
cooked	
10.7 oz (yield from 1 lb)	1,131
4 oz	422
Beef, dried, creamed, home recipe	
8 oz	350
Beef, hearts, lean only	
raw	
8 oz	245

braised	
4 oz	213
1 cup, chopped	273
Beef, kidneys	
raw, 8 oz	294
braised	
4 oz	286
1 cup, chunks	353
Beef, liver	
raw, 1 lb	635
fried, 4 oz	260
Beef pancreas, raw, 4 oz	
fat	358
medium fat	321
lean	160
Beef suet, raw, 1 oz	242
Beef sweetbreads (thymus)	
yearlings, raw, 1 lb	939
yearlings, braised, 4 oz	365
Beef, tongue	
very fat, raw, trimmed, 8 oz	615
fat, raw, trimmed, 8 oz	524
medium-fat, raw, trimmed	
8 oz	470
braised, 4 oz	277
Beef, tripe, 4 oz	
commercial	113
pickled	70

Lamb, fresh

Leg, lean with fat	
raw, with bone, 1 lb	845
roasted, with bone	
9.4 oz (yield from 1 lb)	745
raw, boneless, 1 lb	1,007
roasted, boneless	
11.2 oz (yield from 1 lb)	887
4 oz	317
1 cup, chopped	391
Leg, lean	
roasted, with bone	
7.8 oz (yield from 1 lb with fat)	411
roasted, boneless	
9.7 oz (yield from 1 lb with fat)	491
4 oz	211
1 cup, chopped	260
Loin chops, with bone, lean with fat	
raw, 1 lb	1,146
broiled	
10.1 oz (yield from 1 lb)	1,023
4 oz	407
1 chop, 3.4 oz	341
1 chop, 2.5 oz	255
Loin chops, with bone, lean only	
broiled	
6.9 oz (yield from 1 lb)	368
4 oz	213
1 chop, 2.3 oz	122

1 chop, 1.7 oz	92
Rib chops with bone, lean with fat	
raw, 1 lb	1,229
broiled	
9.5 oz (yield from 1 lb)	1,091
4 oz	462
1 chop, 3.1 oz	362
1 chop, 2.4 oz	273
Rib chops with bone, lean only	
broiled	
6 oz (yield from 1 lb)	361
4 oz	239
1 chop, 2 oz	120
1 chop, 1.5 oz	91
Shoulder, lean with fat	
raw with bone, 1 lb	1,082
roasted, with bone	
9.5 oz (yield from 1 lb)	913
raw, boneless, 1 lb	1,275
roasted, boneless	
11.2 oz (yield from 1 lb)	1,075
4 oz	383
1 cup, chopped	473
Shoulder, lean only	
roasted, with bone	
7 oz (yield from 1 lb)	410
roasted, boneless	
8.3 oz (yield from 1 lb)	482
4 oz	233
1 cup, chopped	287

Lamb's quarters	
raw, trimmed, 1 lb	195
boiled, drained	
4 oz	36
1 cup	64
Lamb hearts	
raw, 8 oz	368
braised	
4 oz	295
1 cup, chopped	377
Lamb kidneys	
raw, 8 oz	238
Lamb liver	
raw, 1 lb	617
broiled, 4 oz	296
Lamb tongue	
raw, trimmed, 8 oz	452
braised, 4 oz	288
Lamb sweetbreads (thymus), 4 oz	
raw	106
braised	200

Ham, retail cuts (see also Pork)

Boiled, 8 oz (about 8 slices)	531
Fresh, lean with fat	
raw, 1 lb with bone and skin	1,188

baked	
9.2 oz (yield from 1 lb)	980
raw, 1 lb without bone and skin	1,397
baked	
10.9 oz (yield from 1 lb)	1,152
4 oz	424
1 cup, chopped	524
1 cup, ground	411
Fresh, lean only	
baked, with bone and skin	
6.8 oz (yield from 1 lb)	421
baked, without bone and skin	
8.1 oz (yield from 1 lb with fat)	495
4 oz	246
1 cup, chopped	304
1 cup, ground	239
Light-cured, lean with fat	
raw, with bone and skin, 1 lb	1,100
baked, with bone and skin	
11.3 oz (yield from 1 lb)	925
raw, without bone and skin, 1 lb	1,279
baked, without bone and skin	
13.1 oz (yield from 1 lb)	1,075
4 oz	328
1 cup, chopped	405
1 cup, ground	318
Light-cured, lean only	
baked, with bone and skin	
8.7 oz (yield from 1 lb with fat)	460

baked, without bone and skin
10.2 oz (yield from 1 lb with fat) 539
baked, without bone and skin
4 oz 328
1 cup, chopped 405
1 cup, ground 318
Long-cured, dry, unbaked
medium-fat, lean with fat, with bone and skin, 4 oz 384
lean, lean with fat, with bone and skin, 4 oz 302
Ham, minced, 4 oz 259

Pork, fresh

Boston butt, shoulder, with bone and skin, lean with fat
raw, 1 lb 1,220
roasted, 10.2 oz (yield from 1 lb) 1,024
Boston butt, shoulder, without bone and skin, lean with fat
raw, 1 lb 1,302
roasted
10.9 oz (yield from 1 lb) 1,087
1 cup, chopped 494
1 cup, ground 388
Boston butt, shoulder, with bone and skin, lean only
roasted, 8.1 oz (yield from 1 lb with fat) 559

Boston butt, shoulder, without bone and skin, lean only	
roasted	
8.6 oz (yield from 1 lb with fat)	595
1 cup, chopped	342
1 cup, ground	268
Loin chops, with bone, lean with fat	
raw, 1 lb	1,065
broiled	
8.2 oz (yield from 1 lb)	911
1 chop, 2.7 oz	305
1 chop, 2 oz	227
Loin chops without bone, lean with fat	
raw, 1 lb	1,352
broiled	
10.4 oz (yield from 1 lb)	1,153
4 oz	411
Loin chops, with bone, lean only	
broiled	
5.9 oz (yield from 1 lb with fat)	454
1 chop, 2 oz	151
1 chop, 1.5 oz	113
Loin chops, without bone, lean with fat	
raw, 1 lb	1,065
baked or roasted, 8.6 oz (yield from 1 lb)	883
Loin roast, without bone, lean with fat	
raw, 1 lb	1,352
baked or roasted	
10.9 oz (yield from 1 lb)	1,115
4 oz	411
1 cup, chopped	507

Loin roast, with bone, lean only	
baked or roasted	
6.9 oz (yield from 1 lb with fat)	495
1 cup, chopped	356
Loin roast, without bone, lean only	
baked or roasted	
8.7 oz (yield from 1 lb with fat)	627
4 oz	288
1 cup, chopped	356
Picnic, shoulder, with bone and skin, lean with fat	
raw, 1 lb	1,083
simmered, 8.4. oz (yield from 1 lb)	890
Picnic, shoulder, without bone and skin, lean with fat	
raw, 1 lb	1,315
simmered	
10.2 oz (yield from 1 lb)	1,085
4 oz	424
1 cup, chopped	524
Picnic, shoulder, with bone and skin, lean only	
simmered, 6.2 oz (yield from 1 lb with fat)	373
Picnic, shoulder, without bone and skin, lean only	
simmered	
7.6 oz (yield from 1 lb with fat)	456
4 oz	241
1 cup, chopped	297
Spareribs, with bone, lean with fat	
raw, 1 lb	976
braised	
6.3 oz (yield from 1 lb)	792
4 oz	499

Pork, specialty cuts, hog

Hearts	
raw, 4 oz	128
braised, 4 oz	221
braised, 1 cup	283
Kidneys, raw, 8 oz	240
Liver	
raw, 1 lb	594
fried, 4 oz	205
Pancreas (Sweetbreads), 4 oz	274
Spleen, raw, 4 oz	122
Tongue, 4 oz	
raw, trimmed	244
braised	287

Pork, specialty cuts, pig, 4 oz

Feet, pickled	227
Salt Pork	
with skin	1,137
without skin	888
Stomach, scalded	274

Pork, cured, retail shoulder cuts (for other cured cuts see Bacon and Ham)

Boston butt, with bone and skin, lean with fat	
unbaked, 1 lb	1,277
baked or roasted, 11 oz (yield from 1 lb)	1,030
Boston butt, without bone and skin, lean with fat	
unbaked, 1 lb	1,320
baked or roasted	
11.8 oz from 1 lb	1,109
4 oz	374
1 cup, chopped	462
1 cup, ground	363
Boston butt, with bone and skin, lean only	
baked or roasted, 9.1 oz (yield from 1 lb with fat)	629
Boston butt without bone and skin, lean only	
baked or roasted	
9.8 oz (yield from 1 lb with fat)	678
4 oz	276
1 cup, chopped	340
1 cup, ground	267
Picnic, with bone and skin, lean with fat	
unbaked, 1 lb	1,060
baked or roasted, 9.7 oz (yield from 1 lb)	888
Picnic, without bone and skin, lean with fat	
unbaked, 1 lb	1,293
baked or roasted	
11.8 oz (yield from 1 lb)	1,085
4 oz	366
1 cup, chopped	452

1 cup, ground	355
Picnic, with bone and skin, lean only	
baked or roasted, 6.8 oz (yield from 1 lb with fat)	405
Picnic, without bone and skin, lean only	
baked or roasted	
8.3 oz (yield from 1 lb with fat)	496
4 oz	239
1 cup, chopped	295
1 cup, ground	232
Bacon, Canadian	
uncooked, 1 lb	980
fried, drained	
12 oz (approx. yield from 1 lb)	921
4 oz	311
1 slice 3⅜" wide	58
Bacon, cured	
raw, 1 lb	3,016
fried, drained	
5.1 oz (approx. yield from 1 lb)	860
1 thick slice	72
1 medium slice	43
1 thin slice	30

Veal, fresh, retail cuts

Chuck cuts and boneless for stew, lean with fat	
raw, with bone, 1 lb	628
stewed, with bone, 8.4 oz (yield from 1 lb)	564

raw, without bone, 1 lb	785
stewed, without bone	
10.6 oz (yield from 1 lb)	703
4 oz	267
1 cup, chopped	329
Loin cuts, lean with fat	
raw, with bone, 1 lb	681
braised, or broiled, with bone	
9.5 oz (yield from 1 lb)	629
raw, without bone, 1 lb	821
braised or broiled, without bone	
11.4 oz (yield from 1 lb)	758
4 oz	245
1 cup, chopped	328
Plate (breast of veal), lean with fat	
raw, with bone, 1 lb	828
braised or stewed, with bone,	
8.3 oz (yield from 1 lb)	718
raw, without bone, 1 lb	1,048
braised or stewed, without bone	
10.6 oz (yield from 1 lb)	906
4 oz	344
Rib roast, lean with fat	
raw, with bone, 1 lb	723
roasted, with bone, 8.5 oz (yield from 1 lb)	648
raw, without bone, 1 lb	939
roasted, without bone	
11 oz (yield from 1 lb)	842
4 oz	305
1 cup, chopped	377

1 cup, ground 296
Round with rump (roasts and leg cutlets), lean with fat
raw, with bone, 1 lb 573
braised or broiled, with bone
8.7 oz (yield from 1 lb) 534
raw, without bone, 1 lb 744
braised or broiled, without bone
11.3 oz (yield from 1 lb) 693
4 oz 245
1 cup, chopped 302

Veal, specialty cuts

Calf hearts
raw, 4 oz 140
braised, 4 oz 236
1 cup 302
Calf kidneys, raw, 8 oz 256
Calves' liver
raw, 4 oz 212
fried, 4 oz 296
Calf pancreas, 4 oz, raw 183
Calf tongue, 4 oz
raw, trimmed 143
braised 181
Calf sweetbreads (thymus), 4 oz
raw 106
braised 192

7 Cold Cuts, Sausages and other meats

Beaver, roasted, 8 oz.	563
Bockwurst	
1 lb (approx 7 links)	1,198
1 link (approx 2.3 oz)	172
Bologna	
without binders	
chub, 1 slice (3″ x ⅛″)	36
ring, 12 oz ring (15″ x 1⅜″)	942
sliced, 1 slice (approx 1 oz)	79
with cereal	
chub, 1 slice	34
ring, 12 oz ring	891
sliced, 1 slice	74
Brains, all types, fresh, raw, 8 oz	284
Capicola	
1 oz	141
1 slice	105
Cervelat, dry	
1 oz	128
4 slices	54
Frankfurter's without binders	
1 lb	1,343
1 frank (5″ x ¾″)	133
Frog's legs, raw	
whole, with bone, 1 lb	215
meat only, 4 oz	83
Meat Loaf, 4 oz	227

Muskrat, roasted, 4 oz	174
Rabbit, domesticated	
raw, whole, ready to cook, 1 lb	581
raw, meat only, 4 oz	184
stewed	
whole 8.6 oz (yield from 1 lb)	529
meat only	
4 oz	245
1 cup, chopped	302
1 cup, ground	238
Rabbit, wild	
whole, ready to cook, 1 lb	490
meat only, 4 oz	153
Raccoon, roasted, meat only, 4 oz	290
Reindeer, raw, lean meat only, 4 oz	144
Salami	
dry roll	
8¼ oz roll	1,053
1 slice	23
dry slice	
4 oz	509
1 slice	45
cooked	
8 oz	706
1 slice approx 1 oz	88
Sausage	
Blood pudding	
4 oz	447
1 slice	32

Polish	
4 oz	345
pork, raw	
2 oz patty	284
1 oz link (4″ x 7/8″)	141
pork, cooked	
4 oz	543
1 patty	129
1 link	62
scrapple	
4 oz	244
1 slice (9/10 oz)	54
souse	
4 oz	205
1 slice (1 oz)	51
Sheep tongue	
raw, trimmed, 8 oz	602
braised, 4 oz	366
Snails, raw, 4 oz	
meat only	103
Giant African, meat only	83
Spleen, all types, 4 oz	125
Terrapin (diamondback), raw	
in shell, 1 lb	106
meat only, 4 oz	126
Thuringer cervelat (summer sausage)	
8 oz	697
1 slice (approx 1 oz)	87
Turtle, green, raw	
in shell, 1 lb	97

meat only, 4 oz	101
Venison, raw, lean meat only, 4 oz	143

MEAT, COMMERCIALLY PACKAGED

Cured and processed meat, 1 oz unless noted

Bacon, cooked, 1 slice	
Hormel	
Black Label	35
Range Label	45
Red Label	37
Oscar Mayer	40
Swift	40
Bacon bits	
Wilson	140
Beef, chopped	
Eckrich, 1 slice	40
Wilson	91
Beef, corned	
Dinty Moore	65
Libby's	101
Safeway	35

Beef, corned brisket	
Swift	80
Wilson	45
Beef, dried	
Swift	42
Beef, roast	
Wilson	33
Beef, smoked	
Safeway	35
spicy	40
Beef steaks	
Hormel	92
Bologna, 1 slice	
Eckrich	90
thick-sliced	160
Hormel	95
Swift	87
Wilson	87
Beef bologna	
Eckrich	95
Beef Smorgas	70
Oscar Mayer	70
Coarse ground bologna	
Hormel	75
Fine ground bologna	
Hormel	80
Garlic bologna	
Eckrich	95
Braunschweiger	
Oscar Mayer	100

Wilson	90
Frankfurters, 1 frank	
Eckrich	120
Jumbo	190
Skinless	150
Hormel	180
Wieners	105
Oscar Mayer	140
Wilson	140
Beef frankfurters, 1 frank	
Eckrich	150
Jumbo	190
Hormel	
Wieners	105
Wranglers	160
Oscar Mayer	140
Vienna	130
Wilson	136
Ham, lunch meat	
cooked	
Eckrich, 1 slice	40
Hormel	35
Safeway	50
Oscar Mayer, 1 slice	30
chopped	
Hormel	70
Oscar Mayer, 1 slice	65
chopped, smoked	
Eckrich	40

Ham, whole, canned, 1 oz	
Amber	110
Oscar Mayer	32
Swift	63
Wilson	
boned and rolled	56
fully cooked	48
Tender Made	44
Ham, whole, packaged, 1 oz	
Hormel	
bone-in	52
Cure 82	48
Curemaster	35
Oscar Mayer	36
Swift	43
Wilson	48
Ham steaks, 1 slice	
Oscar Mayer	70
Ham patties, 1 patty	
Hormel	200
Swift	250
Ham and Cheese Loaf, 1 slice	
Oscar Mayer	75
Honey Loaf, 1 slice	
Eckrich	45
Oscar Mayer	40
Liver, beef	
Swift	54
Liver cheese, 1 slice	
Oscar Mayer	110

Old Fashioned Loaf, 1 slice	
Eckrich	75
Oscar Mayer	65
Olive Loaf, 1 slice	
Oscar Mayer	65
Pastrami, 1 slice	
Eckrich	47
Safeway	40
Pepperoni	
Hormel	140
Swift	150
Pickle Loaf, 1 slice	
Eckrich	85
Oscar Mayer	65
Polish Sausage	
Eckrich	100
Frito-Lay	73
Hormel	80
Pork Butt	
Wilson	72
Pork Loin	
Eckrich	47
Pork Steaks	
Hormel	73
Salami	
Hormel	327
Oscar Mayer, 1 slice	50
Sausage, beef	
Eckrich	95

Sausage, pork	
Hormel	95
Wilson	135
Sausage links, 1 sausage	
Hormel	
Brown 'n Serve	78
Little Sizzlers	67
Midget Links	112
Oscar Mayer	65
Swift	75
Sausage links, smoked, 1 sausage	
Eckrich	190
skinless	115
Smok-Y-Links	75
Hormel	92
Oscar Mayer	140
Scrapple	
Oscar Mayer	45
Sizzlean	
Swift	50
Spam	
Hormel	85
Summer Sausage	
Swift	90
Thuringer	
Hormel	100
Tripe	
Libby's canned	35

Veal Steaks	
Hormel	35
breaded	60
Vienna Sausage, 1 sausage	
Hormel	52
Libby's	84
with barbecue sauce	76

Canned Meat Entrees, 1 can, various sizes

Beef with barbecue sauce	
Morton House	240
Beef, corned with cabbage	
Hormel	150
Beef Goulash	
Hormel	240
Beef sliced with gravy	
Morton House	190
Chili con carne	
Hormel	340
Libby's	130
Morton House	340
Chili con carne with beans	
A&P	440
Hormel	320
Libby's	180
Morton House	340
Swanson	310
Hash, beef with potatoes	
Dinty Moore	270

Item	Calories
Hash, corned beef	
Ann Page	400
Armour Star	435
Bounty	405
Broadcast	480
Libby's	160
Morton House	480
Wilson	480
Hash, roast beef	
Hormel	375
Meatballs in gravy	
Chef Boy-Ar-Dee	315
Pork, sliced with gravy	
Morton House	190
Salisbury Steak with mushroom gravy	
Morton House	160
Sloppy Joe	
Banquet	250
Gebhardt	280
Hormel	365
Libby's	
beef	163
pork	139
Stew, beef	
Armour Star	200
B & M	163
Bounty	213
Dinty Moore	184
Heinz	253
Morton House	312

James River Smithfield	186
Libby's	78
Morton House	240
Swanson	190
Wilson	202
Stew, lamb	
B & M	247
Stew, meatball	
Chef Boy-Ar-Dee	218
Libby's	121
Morton House	290
Stew, Mulligan	
Dinty Moore	240

Frozen Meat Entrees, 1 whole package, various sizes (see also pp 385-391, Frozen Dinners)

Beef	
Banquet	
Cookin' Bag	124
Buffet Supper, 32 oz	782
Green Giant Boil-in-Bag	130
Seabrook Farms	263
Stouffer's	235
Swanson	190
Swanson Hungry-Man	330

Beef goulash	
Seabrook Farms	198
Beef Pot Pie	
Banquet	412
Swanson	443
Beef Stroganoff	
Stouffer's	390
Green Pepper Steak	
Stouffer's	350
Meat Loaf	
Banquet	
Buffet Supper, 32 oz	1,445
Cookin' Bag	224
Man Pleaser	916
Morton	430
Swanson	330
Noodles and Beef	
Banquet Buffet Supper, 32 oz	754
Salisbury Steak	
Banquet	873
Green Giant Boil-in-Bag	390
Morton	490
Stouffer's	500
Swanson	370
Swanson Hungry-Man	640
Salisbury Steak with gravy	
Banquet	
Buffet Supper, 32 oz	1,454
Cookin' Bag	246

Green Giant Oven Bake	290
Sausage, cheese, and tomato pie	
Weight Watchers	390
Sloppy Joe	
Banquet Cookin' Bag	199
Green Giant Boil-in-Bag	160
Steak	
Weight Watchers	390
Stew, Beef	
Banquet Buffet Supper, 32 oz	700
Green Giant Boil-in-Bag	160
Lambrecht	432
Seabrook Farms	229
Stouffer's	310
Stuffed Cabbage with beef	
Green Giant Oven Bake	220
Stuffed Green Pepper with Beef	
Green Giant Oven Bake	200

Meat Substitutes, 1 piece or slice

Morningstar Farms	
Breakfast Links	62
Breakfast Patties	111
Breakfast Strips	38

Loma Linda

Bologna	190
Burgers	
Redi-Burger	150
Sizzle Burger	180
Frankfurters	110
Linketts	70
Little Links	45
Meatballs	48
Peanut Butter	
Nuteena	210
Proteena	160
Roast Beef	200
Salami	210
Sausage	
Breakfast Links	50
Breakfast Sausage	140
Swiss Steak	140
Tender Bits	20
Tender Rounds	50
Turkey	190
Vegeburger, 1 cup	240
Vegelona	160

POULTRY, FRESH

Chickens, fresh

Broilers	
broiled, with skin, giblets	
7.1 oz (yield from 1 lb)	273
meat only, 4 oz	154
Capon, raw, ready to cook, 1 lb	382
Fryers	
raw, ready to cook, 1 lb	382
fried, with skin, giblets	
8 oz (yield from 1 lb)	565
fried, without skin	
dark meat, 4 oz	249
light meat, 4 oz	223
1 back (approx 2 oz)	139
½ breast (approx 3.3 oz)	160
1 drumstick (approx 2 oz)	88
1 neck (approx 2 oz)	127
½ rib section (approx ¾ oz)	41
1 thigh (approx 2.3 oz)	122
1 wing (approx 1.8 oz)	82
skin only (approx 1 oz)	119
Roasters	
raw, ready to cook, 1 lb	791
roasted, with skin, giblets	
8.4 oz (yield from 1 lb)	576

roasted, without skin, dark meat	
4 oz	204
1 cup, chopped	258
1 cup, ground	202
roasted, without skin, light meat	
4 oz	207
1 cup, chopped	255
1 cup, ground	200
Stewing hens or cocks	
raw, ready to cook, 1 lb	987
stewed, with skin, giblets, 8 oz (yield from 1 lb)	708
stewed, without skin, dark meat	
4 oz	235
1 cup, chopped	290
1 cup, ground	228
stewed, without skin, light meat	
4 oz	204
1 cup, chopped	252
1 cup, ground	198
Chicken gizzards	
raw, 1 lb	513
simmered	
12 oz (yield from 1 lb)	497
4 oz	168
1 cup, chopped	215
Chicken hearts	
raw, 4 oz	152
simmered	
4 oz	221
1 cup, chopped	283

Chicken liver	
raw, 1 lb	585
simmered	
4 oz	187
1 cup, chopped	231
1 liver 2" x 2" x ½"	45

Duck, fresh

Domesticated	
raw, meat only, 4 oz	188
roasted, meat only, 4 oz	352
Wild	
raw, meat only, 4 oz	157

Goose, fresh, domesticated

raw, whole, ready to cook, 1 lb	1,172
roasted	
whole, 8½ oz (yield from 1 lb)	1,022
meat only, 4 oz	266
meat and skin, 4 oz	503
Goose gizzards, raw, 1 lb	631
Goose liver, raw, 1 lb	826

Pheasant, fresh

raw, ready to cook, whole, 1 lb	596
raw, meat only, 4 oz	184

Quail, fresh, raw

whole, ready to cook, 1 lb	686
meat and skin only, 4 oz	196
giblets, 2 oz	100

Squab (Pigeon), fresh, raw

whole, dressed, 1 lb	569
meat only, 4 oz	162
light meat only, 4 oz	143

Turkey, fresh

raw, whole, ready to cook, 1 lb	722
roasted, whole, with giblets and skin 8.6 oz (yield from 1 lb)	644
roasted, dark meat without skin 4 oz	230

1 cup, chopped	284
1 cup, ground	223
roasted, light meat without skin	
4 oz	200
1 cup, chopped	246
1 cup, ground	194
roasted, skin only, 1 oz	256
giblets	
raw, 4 oz	170
simmered	
4 oz	254
1 cup, chopped	338
gizzards	
raw, 1 lb	712
simmered	
12 oz (yield from 1 lb)	659
4 oz	222
1 cup, chopped	284
hearts	
raw, 4 oz	169
simmered	
4 oz	245
1 cup, chopped	313
liver	
raw, 1 lb	626
simmered	
4 oz	197
1 cup, chopped	244

7 POULTRY, COMMERCIALLY CANNED, FROZEN, OR PACKAGED: 1 package, various sizes, unless noted (see also pp 385-391, Frozen Dinners)

Chicken

a la King	
Banquet	138
Green Giant	170
Lambrecht	585
Stouffer's	330
Swanson	190
Boned	
Hormel	110
Richardson & Robbins	328
Swanson	110
Chopped, 1 slice	
Eckrich	47
Cacciatore	
Seabrook Farms	248
Creamed	
Stouffer's	300

Creole
Weight Watchers 250
Croquette
Howard Johnson's 505
Divan
Stouffer's 335
and Dumplings
Banquet 282
Morton House, 8 oz 363
Swanson 230
Escalloped
Stouffer's 500
Fricasse, 1 cup
College Inn 240
Richardson & Robbins 229
Fried
Banquet 259
Morton 600
Swanson 290
Livers with broccoli
Weight Watchers 220
with Noodles
Banquet 764
Green Giant 250
Howard Johnson 384
Heinz 186
Pot Pie
Banquet 412
Morton 318
Stouffer's 545

Swanson	430
Swanson Hungry-Man	770
with Rice	
Morton House, 8 oz	460
Smoked	
Safeway, 1 oz	50
Stew, 8 oz	
B & M	168
Bounty	221
Libby's	88
Swanson, 7½ oz	180
White meat with peas and onions	
Weight Watchers	270

Turkey

Boned	
Hormel	90
with Giblet gravy	
Banquet	128
Banquet Buffet Supper	170
Pot Pie	
Banquet	415
Morton	390
Stouffer's	460
Swanson	430
Swanson Hungry-Man	770

Slices	
Banquet	98
Banquet Buffet Supper	564
Green Giant	100
Morton Country Table	390
Morton House canned	140
Swanson	260
Swanson Hungry-Man	380
Tetrazzini	
Stouffer's	480
Smoked	
Eckrich, 1 slice	47
Safeway, 1 oz	50

SEAFOOD, FRESH,
4 oz unless noted

Abalone, raw	
in shell	47
meat only	111
Barracuda, Pacific, raw	
meat only	129
Bass, black sea, raw	
whole	41
meat only	106

Bass, all varieties, raw	
whole	51
meat only	120
Blackfish, see Tautug	
Bonito, raw	
meat only	192
Butterfish, raw, meat only	
gulf	108
northern	192
Catfish, raw, fillets	117
Caviar, sturgeon	
granular	
1 oz	74
1 Tbsp	42
pressed	
1 oz	90
1 Tbsp	54
Clams, raw, meat only	
hard or round	
1 pt	363
8 oz	182
4 cherrystones or 5 littlenecks	56
soft	
1 pt	372
8 oz	186
Cod	
raw, fillets, 8 oz	176
broiled, with butter	
1 steak	352

4 oz	192
dehydrated, lightly salted	308
1 cup, shredded	158
dried, salted	148
Crab, steamed, 8 oz	
in shell	100
meat only	211
Crab, deviled	
8 oz	427
Crab, Imperial	
8 oz	334
Crayfish, raw	
in shell	10
meat only	82
Croaker, Atlantic	
raw, meat only	109
Croaker, white	
raw, meat only	95
Croaker, yellow	
raw, meat only	101
Cusk	
raw, meat only	85
steamed, meat only	120
Eulachon, see Smelt	
Finnan Haddie	
meat only	117
Flounder, fillets	
raw	89
baked with butter	229

Grouper, raw	
whole	42
meat only	99
Haddock	
raw	
whole, 1 lb	172
fillets, 1 lb	360
fried, breaded, 4 oz	187
Halibut, Atlantic or Pacific	
raw	
whole, 1 lb	268
fillets, 1 lb	452
broiled with butter, fillets, 4 oz	199
Herring	
Atlantic, raw	
whole, 1 lb	405
meat only, 4 oz	200
Pacific	
raw, meat only, 4 oz	111
salted (in brine), 4 oz	247
smoked, 4 oz	
bloaters	222
hard	340
kippers	239
Inconnu, raw	
whole	104
meat only	166
Kingfish, raw	
whole	52

meat only	119
Lake Herring (Cisco), raw	
whole	55
meat only	110
Lake Trout, raw	
whole	70
meat only	190
Ling Cod, raw	
whole	44
meat only	96
Lobster, northern	
in shell, 1 lb	
raw	107
cooked	112
Mackerel, Atlantic	
raw, 1 lb	
whole	468
fillets	866
broiled with butter, fillets,	
13 oz yield from 1 lb	861
4 oz	268
Mackerel, Pacific, raw	
whole	130
meat only	181
Mackerel, salted	345
Mackerel, smoked	248
Mullet, raw	
whole	88
meat only	166

- **Muskellunge, raw**
  - whole — 60
  - meat only — 124
- **Mussels, Atlantic or Pacific, raw**
  - in shell — 38
  - meat only — 108
- **Ocean Perch, Atlantic**
  - raw
    - whole — 31
    - meat only — 100
  - fried, breaded — 258
- **Ocean Perch, Pacific, raw**
  - whole — 29
  - meat only — 108
- **Octopus, raw** — 83
- **Oysters, raw**
  - Eastern
    - in shell, 1 lb — 30
    - meat only, 4 oz — 75
    - 1 medium — 20
  - Pacific Western
    - meat only, 4 oz — 105
    - 1 medium — 55
- **Oysters, cooked**
  - fried, breaded, 1 medium — 25
- **Pickerel, raw** — 95
- **Perch, raw**
  - white
    - whole — 48
    - meat only — 134

yellow	
whole	40
meat only	103
Pike, raw	
blue	
whole	45
meat only	100
northern	
whole	26
meat only	100
walleye	
whole	60
meat only	105
Pompano, raw	
whole	106
meat only	188
Porgy, raw	52
meat only	127
Rockfish	
raw	110
steamed	115
Roe, raw	
carp, cod, haddock, herring, pike, and shad	148
salmon, sturgeon, and turbot	236
Sablefish, raw	
whole	90
meat only	216
Salmon, raw	
Atlantic	
whole	160

meat only	246
King (Chinook) meat only	252
Salmon, smoked	200
Sand Dab, raw	
meat only	89
Sardines, Pacific	
raw, meat only	180
Sauger, raw	
whole	34
meat only	95
Scallops, meat only	
raw	92
steamed	127
Sea Bass, white	
raw, meat only	109
Shad, raw	
whole	92
meat only	192
Sheepshead, Atlantic, raw	
whole	60
meat only	128
Shrimp	
raw, whole	
in shell	72
shelled	100
fried, breaded	250
Skate	
raw, meat only	111
Smelt, raw	
whole	60

meat only	110
Snapper, Red and Gray, raw	
whole	55
meat only	106
Sole, raw	
whole	29
meat only (fillet)	90
Spanish Mackerel, raw	
whole	142
meat only	200
Spot	
raw, meat only	250
Squid	
raw, meat only	95
Sturgeon, meat only	
raw	105
steamed	180
Sturgeon, smoked	170
Sucker, carp	
raw	48
meat only	125
Sucker, white and mullet, raw	
whole	195
meat only	118
Swordfish, meat only	
raw	138
broiled in butter	185
Tautug (Blackfish), raw	
whole	37
meat only	101

Tilefish
- raw
  - whole 46
  - meat only 90
- baked, meat only 155

Tomcod, raw
- whole 34
- meat only 88

Trout, Brook, raw
- whole 56
- meat only 115

Trout, Rainbow, raw
- meat only 220

Tuna, raw, meat only
- bluefin 165
- yellowfin 150

Turbot, Greenland, raw
- whole 86
- meat only 166

Weakfish
- raw
  - whole 66
  - meat only 138
- broiled in butter 230

Whitefish, raw
- whole 82
- meat only 177
- smoked 177

Wreckfish
- raw, meat only 130

Yellowtail	
raw, meat only	157

SEAFOOD, CANNED AND FROZEN

Catfish, ocean	
Gorton's, 1 pkg	286
Clams	
Doxsee	
6 oz	84
8 oz	112
12 oz	147
Howard Johnson's	
5 oz	395
Croquettes, 1 pkg	608
Mrs. Paul's 1 cake	180
Thins, 1 cake	155
Sticks, 1 stick	48
Sau-Sea, 1 jar	99
Snow's	60
Cod, 1 pkg	
fillets	
Gorton's	355
San Juan	336
Ship Ahoy	336

sticks	
Bird's Eye	552
Gorton's	830
Crab	
Gold Seal, 1 can	185
Icy Point, 1 can	215
Mrs. Paul's, 1 cake	60
Pillar Rock, 1 can	216
Ship Ahoy, 8 oz	210
Wakefield's, 6 oz	160
Crepes, 5½ oz	
Mrs. Paul's	
Clam	280
Crab	240
Scallop	220
Shrimp	250
Croquettes	
Howard Johnson's	
Shrimp with Newburg Sauce	480
Eel, smoked	185
Vita	402
Fish Au Gratin	
Mrs. Paul's 1 pkg	250
Fish cakes, fillets and sticks, 1 piece	
Mrs. Paul's	105
Beach Haven	110
Thins	160
Fish and Chips	
Swanson, 1 pkg	290

Fish Parmesan	
Mrs. Paul's, 1 pkg	220
Flounder	
Mrs. Paul's, 1 pkg	110
Weight Watchers, 1 pkg	160
Gelfilte Fish, 1 oz	
Manischewitz	23
Mother's	14
Rokeach	19
Haddock au Gratin	
Howard Johnson's	315
Haddock fillets	
Gorton's, 1 pkg	360
Mrs. Paul's, 1 piece	115
Haddock with stuffing	
Weight Watchers, 1 pkg	180
Herring, pickled, 1 oz	
Vita	40
Oysters, 1 cup	
Bumblebee	172
Perch, fried, 1 piece	
Mrs. Paul's	125
Perch, ocean with broccoli	
Weight Watchers, 1 pkg	190
Salmon, canned, 1 can	
blueback	
Icy Point	
3¾-oz can	181
7¾-oz can	376

Coho steak
  Icy Point
    3¾-oz can 162
pink
  Del Monte
    7¾-oz can 310
red
  Icy Point
    1-lb. can 775
  Pillar Rock
    3¾-oz can 181
    7¾-oz can 376
red sockeye
  Del Monte
    7¾-oz can 340
  Bumblebee
    1 cup 286

Sardines, 1 oz
Del Monte 44
Underwood
  in mustard sauce 52
  in soya bean oil 62
  in tomato sauce 330

Scallops
Mrs. Paul's, 3½ oz 210

Seafood combination
Mrs. Paul's 510

Shrimp
Bumblebee, 1 can 90

Icy Point, 1 can	148
Pillar Rock, 1 can	148
Mrs. Paul's, 1 oz	57
Sau-Sea, 1 oz	80
Shad Roe	
Bumblebee, 1 can	259
Shrimp and Scallops	
Stouffer's, 1 pkg	400
Sole	
Mrs. Paul's, 4½ oz	160
Ship Ahoy, 1 pkg	310
with peas, mushrooms, and lobster sauce	
Weight Watchers, 1 pkg	200
Tuna, canned in oil, drained	
Bumblebee, 1 cup	334
Chicken of the Sea	
3¼-oz can	224
6½-oz can	447
9¼-oz can	636
12½-oz can	860
Del Monte, 6½-oz can	450
Gold Seal, 5-oz can	278
Icy Point, 5-oz can	278
Pillar Rock, 5-oz can	278
Snow Mist, 5-oz can	278
Van Camp, 6¼-oz can	440
Tuna, canned, solid, in water	
Bumblebee, 1 cup	300
Chicken of the Sea, 7-oz can	216

Tuna, creamed, with peas	
Green Giant Boil-in-Bag	140
Tuna Pot Pies	
Banquet	478
Morton	385
Star Kist	397
Turbot with peas and carrots	
Weight Watchers, 1 pkg	280

CHAPTER 8

Fruits and Vegetables

FRESH FRUITS AND VEGETABLES

Acerolas (West Indian Cherries)	
whole, 1 lb	104
pitted, 4 oz	32
3 cherries	7
Amaranth	
whole, 1 lb	100
leaves only, 1 lb	160
Apples	
with skin	
1 lb	242

1 apple (3¼″, 2 per lb)	123
1 apple (2¾″, 3 per lb)	80
1 apple (2½″, 4 per lb)	61
chopped, 1 cup	73
pared	
1 apple (3¼″, 2 per lb)	107
1 apple (2¾″, 3 per lb)	70
1 apple (2½″, 4 per lb)	53
chopped, 1 cup	68
Apples, dehydrated	
uncooked	
8 oz	800
1 cup	355
cooked, sweetened	
8 oz	175
1 cup	195
Apples, dried	
uncooked	
8 oz	625
1 cup	234
cooked, unsweetened	
8 oz	177
1 cup	199
cooked, sweetened	
8 oz	254
1 cup	314
Apricots	
whole	
1 lb	217
1 apricot	18

pitted, halves	
1 lb	231
1 cup	79
Apricots, dehydrated	
uncooked	
8 oz	755
1 cup	330
cooked, sweetened	
8 oz	271
1 cup	339
Apricots, dried	
uncooked	
8 oz	590
1 cup	340
10 medium halves	90
cooked, unsweetened, with liquid	
8 oz	195
1 cup	210
cooked, sweetened, 1 cup	329
Artichokes	
raw, whole, 1 lb	85
boiled, drained, 1 whole bud	67
Asparagus	
raw	
whole, 1 lb	66
cuts, 1 cup	35
boiled, drained	
1 medium spear	3
cuts, 1 cup	29

Avocados, California	
whole, 1 lb	589
peeled and pitted, 1 average	370
diced, 1 cup	260
mashed, 1 cup	390
Avocados, Florida	
whole, 1 lb	389
peeled and pitted, 1 average	200
diced, 1 cup	190
mashed, 1 cup	300
Bamboo shoots, raw	
8 oz	61
1 cup, cuts	40
Bananas	
whole	
1 large (10″)	119
1 medium (9″)	103
1 small (8″)	83
1 cup	
sliced	135
mashed	190
Bananas, dehydrated	
flakes, 1 cup	340
Bananas, red	
whole, 1 average (7¼″)	118
sliced, 1 cup	135
Bean Sprouts, mung	
uncooked	
8 oz	80
1 cup	37

boiled, drained	
8 oz	65
1 cup	35
Bean sprouts, soy	
uncooked	
8 oz	105
1 cup	48
boiled, drained	
8 oz	86
1 cup	48
Beet greens	
raw, trimmed, 1 lb	61
boiled, drained	
8 oz	41
1 cup	26
Beets	
raw, trimmed	
1 lb	137
whole, 1 beet (2″)	21
diced, 1 cup	58
boiled, drained	
whole, 1 beet	16
diced, 1 cup	58
sliced, 1 cup	66
Blackberries	
1 lb	250
1 cup	84
Blueberries	
1 lb	260
1 cup	90

Broccoli	
raw	
whole, 1 lb	90
trimmed, 1 lb	145
boiled, drained	
8 oz	59
1 average stalk 6½ oz	47
cuts, 1 cup	40
Brussel Sprouts	
raw	
whole, 1 lb	200
trimmed, 1 lb	190
boiled, drained	
8 oz	82
1 cup	55
1 average sprout	7
Cabbage, Chinese (Celery Cabbage), raw	
whole, 1 lb	62
trimmed, 1 lb	65
cuts, 1 cup	11
strips, 1 cup	8
Cabbage, green	
raw	
whole, 1 lb	98
trimmed, 1 lb	110
chopped, 1 cup	22
sliced, 1 cup	17
ground, 1 cup	36
boiled, drained, 1 cup	30
Cabbage, dehydrated, 1 oz	87

Cabbage, red, raw	
whole, 1 lb	127
trimmed, 1 lb	141
sliced, 1 cup	22
Cabbage, savoy, raw	
whole, 1 lb	98
trimmed, 1 lb	109
sliced, 1 cup	17
Cabbage, spoon (Bakchoy)	
raw	
whole, 1 lb	73
trimmed, 1 lb	70
cuts, 1 cup	11
boiled, drained, cuts, 1 cup	24
Cantaloupe	
one 5-inch melon	95
cubed, 1 cup	48
Carambola, raw	
whole, 1 lb	150
peeled and seeded, 8 oz	80
Carissas (Natal plums), raw	
whole, 1 lb	273
peeled and seeded, 8 oz	155
sliced, 1 cup	105
Carrot	
raw	
whole, 1 lb	156
whole scraped	
8 oz	95
1 medium	21

diced, 1 cup	60
slices, 1 cup	53
boiled, drained, 1 cup	45
Carrot, dehydrated, 1 oz	100
Casaba melon	
whole	61
cubed, 1 cup	45
Cauliflower	
raw	
whole, 1 lb	48
flowerets	
1 lb	120
1 cup	27
chopped, 1 cup	30
boiled, drained, 1 cup	29
Celeriac root, raw	
whole, 1 lb	155
pared, 1 root approx 1 oz	11
Celery	
raw	
whole, 1 lb	58
1 large outer stalk (8″)	7
1 small inner stalk (5″)	3
chopped, 1 cup	20
boiled, drained, 1 cup	22
Chard, Swiss	
raw	
whole, 1 lb	113
1 lb, then trimmed	104

boiled, drained	
leaves and stalks, 1 cup	26
leaves only, 1 cup	32
Chayote	
raw, 1 medium squash	56
Cherimoya, raw	
whole, 1 lb	247
peeled and seeded, 8 oz	215
Cherries	
sour, red	
whole	
1 lb	213
1 cup	60
pitted, 1 cup	90
sweet	
whole	
1 lb	286
1 cup	82
pitted	
1 cup	102
1 average cherry	5
Chervil	
raw, 1 oz	16
Chives, raw	
whole, 1 lb	128
chopped, 1 Tbsp	1
Coconut, raw	
in shell, 1 coconut (4½" and 27 oz)	1,375
shelled, meat only, 4 oz	392

shredded, 1 cup	
loosely packed	277
firmly packed	450
Coconut, dried, shredded	
unsweetened	
4 oz	750
1 cup	622
sweetened	
4 oz	622
1 cup	515
Collards	
raw	
whole, 1 lb	180
leaves only, 1 lb	205
boiled	
leaves only	60
with stems, 1 cup	43
Corn, sweet	
raw, on the cob, 1 lb	240
boiled, drained	
on the cob, 1 ear (5″)	70
kernels, 1 cup	140
Corn Salad, raw	
whole, 1 lb	90
trimmed, 1 lb	95
Crab apples, raw	
whole, 1 lb	280
trimmed	309
Cranberries	
whole, 1 lb	200

without stems, 1 cup	52
chopped, 1 cup	50
Cranberries, dehydrated, 1 oz	100
Cucumber	
1 lb	65
1 average (7½″)	35
sliced, 1 cup	15
Currants	
black	
whole, 1 lb	240
trimmed, 1 cup	60
red or white	
whole, 1 lb	220
trimmed, 1 cup	55
Dandelion greens	
raw, trimmed, 1 lb	205
boiled, drained, 1 cup	
loosely packed	35
firmly packed	70
Dates, domestic	
whole, 1 lb	1,081
pitted, 1 lb	1,243
chopped, 1 cup	488
1 average date	22
Dock (Sorrel)	
raw, whole, 1 lb	89
boiled, drained, 1 cup	38
Eggplant	
raw	
whole, 1 lb	92

diced, 1 cup	50
boiled, drained, 1 cup	38
Elderberries	
whole, 1 lb	310
without stems, 8 oz	160
Endive (French or Belgian) bleached (Chicory)	
trimmed, 1 lb	68
1 head (6″)	8
1 small leave	½
chopped, 1 cup	14
Escarole	
whole, 1 lb	80
large outer leaf	5
small inner leaf	½
chopped, 1 cup	10
Fennel, raw	
whole, 1 lb	120
trimmed, 2 oz	15
Figs, raw	
whole, 1 lb	360
1 medium (2¼″)	40
dried	
8 oz	620
1 medium (2″)	58
Garlic, raw	
whole, 2 oz	68
peeled	
2 oz	80
1 clove	3

Ginger root	
whole, 1 lb	**205**
peeled, 1 oz	**14**
Green (Snap) Beans, 1 cup	**31**
Gooseberries	
1 lb	**177**
1 cup	**59**
Grapefruit	
pink	
whole, 1 lb	**89**
sections, 1 cup	**80**
white	
whole, 1 lb	**86**
sections, 1 cup	**80**
Grapes	
American slipskin: Concord, Delaware, Niagara	
whole, 1 lb	**197**
seeded	
1 cup	**70**
1 grape	**2**
European close skin: Malaga, Muscat, Thompson	
whole, 1 lb	**270**
seeded, 1 cup	**100**
seedless	
1 cup	**107**
1 grape	**3½**
Ground-cherries, raw	
whole, 1 lb	**220**
without husks	
1 lb	**240**
1 cup	**74**
Guava	
whole, 1 lb	**275**
trimmed, 8 oz	**140**
1 average	**58**
Honeydew Melon	
whole, 1 lb	**94**
cubed, 1 cup	**56**

Jack Fruit	
whole, 1 lb	125
peeled and seeded, 8 oz	110
Jujubes (Chinese dates)	
fresh	
whole, 1 lb	444
seeded, 8 oz	238
dried	
whole, 1 lb	1,160
seeded, 8 oz	650
Kale	
raw	
whole, 1 lb	129
without stems, 1 lb	155
leaves only, 4 oz	80
boiled, drained	
1 cup	31
leaves only, 1 cup	44
Kohlrabi	
raw	
whole, 1 lb	96
pared	
8 oz	65
diced, 1 cup	40
boiled, drained, 1 cup	40
Kumquats	
whole, 1 lb	274
trimmed	
8 oz	150

1 medium	12
Leeks, raw	
whole, 1 lb	123
bulb and lower leaf	
8 oz	116
1 medium	17
Lettuce	
Boston	
whole	
1 lb	47
1 head (5″)	23
1 large, 2 medium or 3 small leaves	2
chopped, 1 cup	8
Iceberg	
whole	
1 lb	56
1 head (6″)	70
1 medium leaf	3
chopped, 1 cup	7
Loose Leaf	
whole	
1 lb	52
3 large leaves	15
chopped, 1 cup	10
Romaine or cos	
whole	
1 lb	52
1 leaf	2
chopped, 1 cup	10

Limes	
whole, 1 lb	106
pulp only, 1 lime	19
Loganberries	
whole, 1 lb	267
trimmed	
8 oz	140
1 cup	90
Loqats	
whole, 1 lb	168
seeded	
8 oz	110
1 medium	6
Mangoes, whole	
1 lb	200
1 medium	150
1 cup	110
Mushrooms, raw	
whole, 1 lb	123
chopped, 1 cup	20
Mustard Greens	
raw	
whole	
1 lb	57
trimmed, 8 oz	70
boiled, drained, leaves only	
8 oz	52
1 cup	32
Mustard Spinach (Tendergreens)	
raw, whole, 1 lb	100

Food	Calories
boiled, drained	
8 oz	37
1 cup	30
Nectarines, whole	
1 lb	267
1 medium	88
New Zealand Spinach	
raw, whole, 1 lb	86
boiled, drained	
8 oz	30
1 cup	23
Okra	
raw	
whole, 1 lb	140
trimmed, 8 oz	80
boiled, drained, sliced, 1 cup	45
Onions, mature	
raw	
whole, 1 lb	157
trimmed	
8 oz	85
1 medium	40
chopped, 1 cup	65
chopped, 1 Tbsp	4
grated, 1 cup	90
boiled, drained, 1 cup	60
Onions, young green	
whole, 1 lb	157
bulb and top	
trimmed, 1 lb	164

chopped, 1 cup	36
chopped, 1 Tbsp	2
top only, chopped	
1 cup	27
1 Tbsp	2
Onions, Welsh	
raw	
whole, 1 lb	100
trimmed, 8 oz	78
Oranges	
whole	
1 lb	162
1 medium	64
diced, 1 cup	103
Papaw	
whole	
1 lb	290
1 medium	83
peeled and seeded	
8 oz	185
1 cup	210
Papayas	
whole	
1 lb	120
1 medium	120
peeled and seeded	
8 oz	90
cubed, 1 cup	55

Parsley	
whole, 1 lb	200
chopped	
1 cup	26
1 Tbsp	2
1 sprig	4
Parsnips	
raw, whole, 1 lb	293
boiled, drained	
diced, 1 cup	100
mashed, 1 cup	140
Passion Fruit	
whole	
1 lb	210
1 medium	15
shelled, 8 oz	200
Peaches	
whole, 1 lb	150
peeled, 1 medium	38
pared, diced, 1 cup	70
Pears, 1 pear	
Bartlett	200
Bosc	85
D'Anjou	120
Peas, green immature	
raw	
whole, 1 lb	150
shelled	
1 lb	380
1 cup	120

boiled, drained	
8 oz	160
1 cup	115
Peas, mature, dried	
raw	
whole	
1 lb	1,540
1 cup	680
split, uncoated, 1 cup	700
cooked, split, uncoated, 1 cup	230
Pea Pods (Snow Peas)	
whole, 1 lb	228
Pepper, Hot chili, green, raw	
whole, 1 lb	120
seeded, 8 oz	85
Pepper, Hot chili, red	
raw	
whole, 1 lb	400
seeded, 8 oz	145
pods, dried, 1 Tbsp	25
Peppers, Sweet, green, raw	
whole	
1 lb	80
1 pepper, fancy grade large	35
1 pepper, No 1 grade	15
chopped, 1 cup	33
Peppers, Sweet, red, raw	
whole, 1 lb	110
seeded and cored, 8 oz	70
chopped, 1 cup	47

Persimmon	
Japanese or Kaki	
whole, 1 lb	286
seedless, 1 lb	295
trimmed, 1 medium	130
native	
whole	
1 lb	475
1 medium	32
trimmed and seeded, 8 oz	65
Pigeon peas	
raw, whole, 1 lb	210
dried, 8 oz	760
Pineapple	
whole, 1 lb	125
cubed, 1 cup	80
Pitanga (Surinam Cherries)	
whole	
1 lb	187
4 medium	10
pitted, 1 cup	87
Plantains, raw	
whole, 1 lb	390
peeled, 8 oz	270
1 banana (10″)	285
Plums	
Damson	
whole	
1 lb	272

Food	Calories
1 medium	7
pitted, 8 oz	150
Japanese	
whole	
1 lb	205
1 medium	32
pitted, 8 oz	110
Prune type	
whole	
1 lb	320
1 medium	21
pitted, 8 oz	170
Poke Shoot (Pokeberry)	
raw, 1 lb	104
boiled, drained, 1 cup	33
Pomegranate	
whole	
1 lb	194
1 medium	100
Potatoes	
raw	
whole, 1 lb	280
peeled, 1 cup	114
baked in skin	
4 oz	81
1 long	145
boiled in skin	
4 oz	79
1 long	173
1 round	104

boiled, peeled	
4 oz	74
1 cup	100
fried, 4 oz	275
hash brown, 4 oz	260
mashed, with milk and butter	
4 oz	107
1 cup	137
scalloped, with cheese, 4 oz	118
Prickly Pears, raw	
whole, 1 lb	84
peeled and seeded, 8 oz	96
Prunes, dehydrated, uncooked	
8 oz	780
1 cup	344
Pumpkin, raw	
whole, 1 lb	83
pulp only, 8 oz	60
Purslane leaves	
raw, whole, 1 lb	95
boiled, drained, 1 cup	27
Quinces	
whole, 1 lb	158
peeled and seeded, 8 oz	130
Radishes, raw	
whole	
1 lb	49
10 medium	8
sliced, 1 cup	20

Radishes, Oriental	
whole, 1 lb	57
without tops, 1 lb	67
pared, 8 oz	45
Raisins, seedless	
8 oz	655
1 cup loose	420
1 cup firmly packed	477
Raspberries	
black	
1 lb	330
1 cup	98
red	
1 lb	260
1 cup	70
Rhubarb	
raw	
whole, 1 lb	33
trimmed, 1 lb	60
diced, 1 cup	20
cooked, sweetened, 1 cup	381
Rose Apples	
whole, 1 lb	170
trimmed and seeded, 8 oz	138
Rutabagas	
raw	
whole, 1 lb	177
trimmed, 8 oz	105
diced, 1 cup	60

boiled, drained	
cubes, 1 cup	60
mashed, 1 cup	84
Sapodillas	
whole, 1 lb	323
peeled and seeded, 8 oz	202
Shallots, raw	
whole, 1 oz	18
peeled	
1 oz	20
1 Tbsp	7
Soursop, raw	
whole, 1 lb	200
peeled and seeded, 8 oz	149
Soybean curd (Tofu)	
4 oz	82
Spinach	
raw	
whole, 1 lb	85
trimmed	
leaves, 1 cup	9
chopped, 1 cup	14
boiled, drained, leaves, 1 cup	41
Squash, summer	
raw	
whole, 1 lb	85
trimmed, 8 oz	25
diced, 1 cup	35
boiled, drained, 1 cup	30

Squash, winter	
raw, whole, 1 lb	150
baked, 8 oz	120
Strawberries, whole	
1 lb	161
trimmed, 1 lb	168
1 cup	55
Sugar Apples (Sweetsop)	
whole, 1 lb	192
peeled and seeded	
8 oz	220
1 cup	235
Swamp Cabbage	
raw	
whole, 1 lb	107
trimmed, 1 lb	132
boiled, drained, 8 oz	48
Sweet Potatoes	
raw, whole, 1 lb	420
baked in skin, 4 oz	125
Tamarinds	
whole, 1 lb	520
shelled and seeded, 8 oz	540
Tomatoes, green	
whole, 1 lb	99
Tomatoes, ripe	
raw	
whole	
1 lb	100
1 medium	25

Food	Calories
sliced, 1 cup	40
boiled, 1 cup	63
Towel Gourd	
whole, 1 lb	70
pared, 8 oz	40
Turnip Greens	
raw	
whole, 1 lb	107
trimmed, 1 lb	127
boiled	
8 oz	46
1 cup	30
Turnips	
raw	
whole, 1 lb	117
cubed, 1 cup	39
boiled, drained	
8 oz	52
1 cup	36
mashed	53
Vinespinach (Basella), raw, 8 oz	44
Water Chestnuts, Chinese	
raw, whole, 1 lb	276
Watercress	
whole	
1 lb	80
1 cup	7
chopped, 1 cup	24
Watermelon	
whole, 1 lb	54

1 wedge (4″ x 8″)	110
diced, 1 cup	42
Wax (Yellow) Beans	
1 cup	29
Yam Beans, raw	
whole, 1 lb	225
pared, 8 oz	130
Yams, raw	
whole, 1 lb	395
pared, 4 oz	115
Zucchini (see Summer Squash)	

FRUIT, COMMERCIALLY PACKAGED, CANNED OR FROZEN,

½ cup unless noted

Apples and Apricots	
Mott's	104
Apples and Cherries	
Mott's	110
Apples and Pineapples	
Mott's	127

Apples and Raspberries	
Mott's	105
Applesauce	
Del Monte	85
Mott's	45
S & W	48
Stokely-Van Camp	90
Tillie Lewis	60
Town House	85
Apricots	
Del Monte	100
Libby's	100
Stokely-Van Camp	110
Tillie Lewis	60
Town House	80
Blackberries	
S & W	36
Blueberries	
Seabrook Farms	45
Boysenberries	
S & W	32
Cherries	
Del Monte Light	95
Dark	90
Dark pitted	95
Libby's	100
S & W	50
Stokely-Van Camp	50
Cherries, maraschino	
Vita 1 cherry	20

Cranberry and Orange	
Ocean Spray	100
Cranberry Sauce	
Ocean Spray	90
Currants	
Del Monte	190
Dates	
Bordo	330
Dromedary	397
Dromedary pitted	376
Figs	
Del Monte	100
S & W, 6 figs	49
Fruit Cocktail	
Del Monte	85
Dole	72
Libby's	75
S & W	35
Stokely-Van Camp	95
Tillie Lewis	50
Town House	85
Fruit Salad	
Del Monte	85
Del Monte Tropical	100
Kraft	48
Libby's	90
S & W	35
Stokely-Van Camp	95
Fruits and Peels	
Liberty	388

Grapefruit sections	
Del Monte	45
Kraft	43
S & W	36
Tillie Lewis	45
Mixed Fruit	
Birds Eye	105
Melon Balls	
Birds Eye, 1 pkg	144
Oranges	
Del Monte	75
Kraft	52
S & W	27
Peaches	
Birds Eye	72
Del Monte	85
Highway	70
S & W	25
Scotch Buy	70
Seabrook Farms	105
Stokely-Van Camp	90
Town House, heavy syrup	95
Town House, extra heavy syrup	130
Peaches and Strawberries	
Birds Eye	80
Pears	
Del Monte	80
Libby's	85
Libby's Juice Pack	75
Highway	80

Scotch Buy	70
S & W	28
Stokely-Van Camp	105
Tillie Lewis	50
Pineapple	
Del Monte in juice	70
Del Monte in syrup	95
Dole in juice	65
Dole in syrup	85
S & W	50
Town House in juice	75
Town House in syrup	95
Plums	
Del Monte	95
Libby's	105
S & W	50
Stokely-Van Camp	120
Tillie Lewis	70
Prunes	
Del Monte	115
Heart's Delight	210
Sunsweet	196
Raspberries	
Birds Eye	120
Seabrook Farms	120
Rhubarb	
Birds Eye	138
Strawberries	
Birds Eye	90
Birds Eye slices	145

Seabrook Farms	42
Seabrook Farms slices	140
S & W	20

VEGETABLES, COMMERCIALLY PACKAGED, CANNED OR FROZEN,

1 cup unless noted

Artichoke Hearts	
Birds Eye	53
Asparagus, cuts	
Green Giant	40
Kounty Kist	40
Lindy	39
Stokely-Van Camp	44
Asparagus, Spears	
Del Monte	35
Green Giant	40
Le Sueur	38
S & W	18
Town House	35
Asparagus, frozen	
Birds Eye	61
with Hollandaise Sauce, 1 pkg	290

Green Giant	90
Seabrook Farms	46
Bamboo Shoots	
Chun King	30
La Choy	23
Bean Sprouts	
Chun King	40
La Choy	24
Beets, cut	
Del Monte	70
Libby's	70
Stokely-Van Camp	90
Beets, diced	
Comstock	82
Libby's	70
Stokely-Van Camp	70
Beets, Harvard	
Greenwood	104
Libby's	160
Lord Mott	80
Stokely-Van Camp	160
Beets, pickled	
Del Monte	150
Greenwood	150
Libby's	150
Lord Mott	150
Stokely-Van Camp	190
Town House	145
Beets, sliced	
Del Monte	70

Libby's	70
Lord Mott	50
S & W	56
Stokely-Van Camp	80
Beets, whole	
Del Monte	70
Libby's	70
Stokely-Van Camp	85
Beets, frozen	
Birds Eye	105
Broccoli, frozen	
Birds Eye	25
with cheese	110
in hollandaise	200
Green Giant	30
in butter	90
in cheese sauce	130
with cauliflower and carrots	140
Kounty Kist	30
Seabrook Farms	46
Stouffer's Au gratin	340
Brussels Sprouts	
Birds Eye	30
Green Giant	50
in butter sauce	110
in cheese sauce	170
Kounty Kist	50
Seabrook Farms	76
Cabbage	
Greenwood	150

Lord Mott	120
Carrots, diced	
Comstock	48
Del Monte	61
Libby's	40
S & W	44
Stokely-Van Camp	60
Carrots, sliced	
Birds Eye, in buttersauce	340
in sugar	194
Comstock	35
Del Monte	58
Green Giant, in butter sauce	100
Libby's	42
Lord Mott	50
Stokely-Van Camp	50
Cauliflower	
Birds Eye	61
with cheese sauce	130
Green Giant	30
with cheese sauce	130
Kounty Kist	26
Seabrook Farms	26
Collard Greens	
Birds Eye	30
Seabrook Farms	44
Corn, Yellow, canned	
cream style	
Birds Eye	170
Del Monte	210

Green Giant	210
S & W	168
Stokely-Van Camp	210
liquid pack	
Del Monte	170
Green Giant	160
Kounty Kist	180
Le Sueur	170
Libby's	160
S & W	104
Stokely-Van Camp	180
vacuum pack	
Del Monte	200
Green Giant	160
Kounty Kist	160
Stokely-Van Camp	240
with peppers	
Del Monte	190
Green Giant	150
Corn, Yellow, frozen	
Birds Eye in butter sauce	200
Green Giant in butter sauce	190
with peppers	180
Stouffer's, 1 pkg	465
Corn, White, frozen and canned	
Birds Eye creamed	170
with peas	140
Del Monte creamed	190
kernels	150
Green Giant	130

Kounty Kist	140
Eggplant Parmesan	
Mrs. Paul's	364
Eggplant slices	
Mrs. Paul's	613
Eggplant sticks	
Mrs. Paul's	254
Kale	
Seabrook Farms	60
Mixed Vegetables, canned	
Del Monte	79
La Choy	35
Libby's	78
Stokely-Van Camp	81
Town House	88
Mixed Vegetables, frozen	
Birds Eye	145
Chun King	23
Green Giant	90
Kounty Kist	89
California	30
La Choy	23
Mixed Vegetables, frozen, Chinese style	
Birds Eye Cantonese	123
Birds Eye International	48
Green Giant	130
La Choy	72
Mixed Vegetables, frozen, European styles	
Birds Eye	
Danish	74

Italian	98
Parisian	74
Mixed Vegetables, frozen, Hawaiian style	
Birds Eye	98
Green Giant	197
Mixed Vegetables, frozen, Japanese style	
Birds Eye	98
Birds Eye with seasonings	74
Green Giant	130
La Choy, 1 pkg	71
Mixed Vegetables, frozen, American styles	
Birds Eye	
New England	150
New Orleans Creole	150
Jubilee	250
Pennsylvania Dutch	98
San Francisco	111
Wisconsin	111
Green Giant	130
Mushrooms	
Birds Eye	50
Brandywine	30
B & B	60
Dole	5
Green Giant	15
Mustard greens	
Birds Eye	44
Seabrook Farms	42
Okra	
Birds Eye	61

Green Giant	211
Seabrook Farms	52
Onions	
Birds Eye	64
in cream sauce	239
whole	98
Green Giant	140
Lord Mott	60
in cream sauce	130
Ore-Ida	80
Seabrook Farms	232
Onion Rings, 1 oz	
Birds Eye	170
Mrs. Paul's	60
O & C	178
Ore-Ida	80
Peas, canned	
early	
Del Monte	110
Kounty Kist	139
Le Sueur	110
Lindy	138
Lord Mott	110
Minnesota Valley	109
Stokely-Van Camp	128
sweet	
Del Monte	101
Green Giant	110
with onion	105
Kounty Kist	131

Libby's	121
Lindy	130
S & W	70
Stokely-Van Camp	130
with carrots	
Del Monte	100
Libby's	101
Lord Mott	165
S & W	65
Stokely-Van Camp	120
Peas, frozen	
early	
Birds Eye	169
Green Giant	102
Kounty Kist	119
Le Sueur	149
Seabrook Farms	148
sweet	
Birds Eye	155
Green Giant	150
Seabrook Farms	104
with carrots	
Birds Eye	122
Kounty Kist	90
Seabrook Farms	82
with cream sauce	
Birds Eye	369
Green Giant	300
with cream sauce and cauliflower	
Birds Eye	247

in onion sauce	
Seabrook Farms	192
with onions	
Birds Eye	149
with onions and carrots	
Le Sueur	180
with potatos	
Birds Eye	431
with mushrooms	
Birds Eye	155
Peppers, green	
Stouffers, 1 pkg	225
Weight Watchers, one 13-oz pkg	320
Potatoes, canned	
Del Monte	90
Hormel au gratin, 7½-oz can	270
with ham, 7½-oz can	255
Stokely-Van Camp	103
Potatoes, frozen, 3 oz unless noted	
Au gratin	
Green Giant, 1 cup	390
Stouffer's	270
French fried	
Birds Eye	
Crinkle Cuts	124
Cottage Fries	120
Gold Crinkle Cuts	140
French	111
Shoestrings	138
Steak Fries	109

Ore-Ida	
Cottage Fries	140
Golden Crinkles	130
Sizzling Fries	157
Sizzling Crinkles	171
Sizzling Shoestrings	218
Shoestrings	170
Hash browns	
Birds Eye	54
O'Brien	45
Ore-Ida	70
in butter sauce	120
in butter sauce and onions	130
with parsley	
Seabrook Farms	208
Scalloped	
Stouffer's	252
Shredded hash browns	
Birds Eye	60
Ore-Ida	60
Slices	
Green Giant	210
with sour cream	
Green Giant	270
Stuffed	
Green Giant	
with cheese, 5 oz	240
with sour cream, 5 oz	229
with peas	
Green Giant	242

Taters and Puffs	
Birds Eye Tasti Fries	140
Tasti Puffs	190
Ore-Ida Tater Tots	160
Tater Tots with Bacon	151
Tater Tots with Onion	165
With Vermicelli	
Green Giant	399
Whole	
Birds Eye	179
Ore-Ida	70
Seabrook Farms	153
Potatoes, mix, ½ cup	
French's	120
Big Tate	129
Hungry Jack	160
Julienne	
Betty Crocker	132
Au gratin	
Betty Crocker	150
French's	190
Creamed	
Betty Crocker	163
Hash browns	
Betty Crocker	147
French's	160
Pancakes	
French's 3 cakes	130
Potato Buds	
Betty Crocker	132

Scalloped
Betty Crocker 150
French's 189
With sour cream
Betty Crocker 144

Pumpkin
Del Monte 79
Libby's 80
Stokely-Van Camp 88

Sauerkraut
Del Monte 50
Libby's 42
Stokely-Van Camp 50
Bavarian 69

Soup Greens
Durkee 213

Spinach, canned
Del Monte 45
Libby's 44
Lord Mott 44

Spinach, frozen
chopped
Birds Eye 47
Seabrook Farms 50
creamed
Birds Eye 157
Green Giant 190
Lord Mott 130

Seabrook Farms	200
leaf	
Birds Eye	47
Seabrook Farms	48
souffle	
Green Giant	300
Stouffer's, 1 pkg	400
with butter sauce	
Green Giant	89
Squash	
Birds Eye	100
Green Giant	118
Seabrook Farms	92
Stew, vegetable	
Dinty Moore, 7½-oz can	160
Ore-Ida	140
Succotash	
Birds Eye	202
Libby's creamed	190
kernel	151
Seabrook Farms	174
Stokely-Van Camp	170
Sweet Potatoes	
Birds Eye	408
Green Giant	341
Lord Mott	235
Mrs. Paul's	320
Tomatoes	
stewed	70
whole	50

Tomato paste	
Contadina	200
Del Monte	200
Hunt's	185
Town House	225
Tomato puree	
Contadina	120
Turnip Greens	
Birds Eye	47
Seabrook Farms	44
Stokely-Van Camp	46
Zucchini	
Birds Eye	39
Del Monte	60
Mrs. Paul's	480

CHAPTER 9

Condiments, Dips, Dressings, Oils and Sauces

CONDIMENTS, 1 Tbsp, unless noted

capers	
Crosse & Blackwell	6
catsup	
Del Monte	15
Heinz	16
Hunt's	18
Smucker's	31
Stokely-Van Camp	21

celery flakes, 1 tsp	
Wyler's	7
curry powder	
Crosse & Blackwell	26
garlic flavoring, 1 tsp	
Burton's	42
garlic powder, 1 tsp	
Wyler's	8
garlic spread	
Lawry's	88
horseradish	
Borden	16
Heinz	26
Kraft	4
Tastee	5
hot sauce, 1 tsp	
Frank's	10
Gebhardt	4
Tabasco	4
meat sauces	
A-1	12
Crosse & Blackwell	21
Durkee	60
Escoffier	19
Gravymaster, 1 tsp	8
Heinz 57	14
Heinz Savory	21
H.P.	21
Maggi	17

Steak Supreme	20
mustard	
Brown	
French's	15
Gulden's	13
Heinz	11
Mr. Mustard	11
Dijon	
Grey Poupon	15
German	
Kraft	15
Horseradish	
French's	15
Hot	
Gulden's Diablo	13
Heinz	11
Onion	
French's	25
Yellow	
French's	16
Gulden's	11
Heinz	10
Kraft	12
onion flakes, 1 tsp	
Wyler's	7
onion flavoring, 1 tsp	
Burton's	42
onion powder, 1 tsp	
Wyler's	1

onions, minced, 1 tsp
- *Borden's* 7
- *Wyler's* 7

parsley flakes, 1 tsp
- *Wyler's* 1

pepper
- Seasoned
  - *Lawry's, 1 tsp* 16
- sweet
  - *Wyler's, 1 tsp* 2

salt, flavored, 1 tsp
- celery 6
- garlic 6
- onion 6

sandwich spread
- *Hellman's* 60
- *Kraft* 56

vinegar
- Cider or white 1
- Wine
  - *Holland House*
    - Marsala 35
    - Red 25
    - Sherry 40
    - White 25
  - *Regina*
    - Sauterne 1
    - Sherry 10

Flavorings, Extracts, 1 tsp

Almond	
Durkee	13
Ehlers	5
Anise	
Durkee	16
Ehlers	12
Banana	
Durkee	15
Ehlers	7
Black Walnut	
Durkee	45
Brandy	
Durkee	15
Ehlers	18
Cherry	
Ehlers	8
Chocolate	
Durkee	8
Coconut	
Durkee	7
Ehlers	13
Lemon	
Durkee	17
Ehlers	14
Maple	
Durkee	6
Ehlers	9

Mocha
Durkee 14
Orange
Durkee 16
Ehlers 14
Peppermint
Durkee 15
Ehlers 12
Pineapple
Ehlers 13
Raspberry
Ehlers 10
Rum
Durkee 14
Ehlers 12
Strawberry
Durkee 12
Ehlers 11
Vanilla
Durkee 5

Relishes, Pickles, Olives: 1 piece unless noted

Capers, 1 Tbsp
Crosse & Blackwell 6

Carrots, dill	
Cresca Cocktail Sticks	1
Cauliflower, sweet	
Heinz	9
Smucker's	23
ChowChow, 1 Tbsp	
Crosse & Blackwell	20
Chutney	
Major Grey's	53
Eggplant	
Cresca	1
Olives	
Green, Manzanilla	
Durkee	4
Grandee	4
Green, Spanish	
Vita	11
Green, queen	
Durkee	14
Grandee	14
Ripe	
Durkee	7
Grandee	7
Lindsay	6
Vita	7
Onions	
Cresca	1
Crosse & Blackwell	1
Heinz	2
Heinz Spiced	1

Peppers, 1 oz unless noted	
Chili	
Del Monte	5
Ortega	
Jalapeños	8
Green	5
Hot, 1 pepper	
Cresca	6
Smucker's	10
Mild, sweet	
Del Monte	5
Pickled	
Old El Paso	9
Red, bell	
Ortega	9
Pickle Relish, 1 Tbsp	
Barbecue	
Crosse & Blackwell	22
Heinz	31
Corn	
Crosse & Blackwell	15
Hamburger	
Crosse & Blackwell	20
Heinz	17
Hot dog	
Crosse & Blackwell	22
Heinz	2
Hot pepper	
Crosse & Blackwell	22

India	
Crosse & Blackwell	26
piccalilli	
Crosse & Blackwell	25
Heinz	19
Pickles	
Sour	
Bond's	2
Crosse & Blackwell	2
Heinz	
Genuine Dill	10
Kosher Dills	2
L & S	2
Sweet	
Bond's	19
Crosse & Blackwell	28
slices, 1 Tbsp	15
Heinz	
Midget	5
Sweet Gherkins	25
Sweet Pickles	45
Sticks	13
Candied dill strips	35
Pimientos, 1 oz	
Dromedary	8
Ortega	7
Stokely-Van Camp	8
Watermelon Rind, 1 Tbsp	38

Seasonings, 1 tsp unless noted

Accent	9
Bacon	
Ann Page	8
Baco's	13
Durkee	3
French's	2
Lawry's	13
McCormick	
Bits	10
Chips	12
Schilling	
Bits	19
Chips	13
Barbecue	
French's	6
Chili Powder	
Lawry's	9
Mexene	8
Cinnamon Sugar	
French's	16
Chutney	
Major Grey's	16
Spice Island	12
Herb	
Lawry's	9
Horseradish	
Reese	18

Hot Sauce	
Frank's	1
Lemon Pepper	
Lawry's	7
French's	6
Meat Tenderizer	
French's	2
Pepper	
French's	8
Lawry's	8
Salad	
Durkee	4
with cheese	10
French's	6
Salt	
French's	
Butter	8
Celery	2
Garlic	4
Hickory Smoked	2
Onion	6
Parsley Garlic	6
Seasoned	2
Lawry's	
Garlic	5
Onion	4
Seasoned	1
Seafood	
French's	2

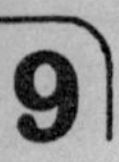

Stock Base	
French's	8

Seasoning Mixes, 1 pkg, various sizes

A la King	
Durkee	297
Beef	
Lawry's	
Beef Olé	126
Marinade	69
Beef Stew	
Durkee	99
French's	150
Lawry's	131
McCormick	90
Schilling	89
Beef Stroganoff	
French's	192
Lawry's	119
McCormick	113
Beef, Ground	
Ann Page	100
Durkee	91
French's	100
Chili	
Ann Page	120
French's	150

Durkee	148
Lawry's	137
McCormick	225
Schilling	226
Chop Suey	
Durkee	128
Enchilada	
Durkee	89
French's	119
Goulash	
Lawry's	127
Hamburger	
Durkee	110
Lipton	30
Meatball	
Durkee	22
with cheese	85
French's	140
Meatloaf	
Contadina	363
French's	160
Lawry's	333
McCormick	120
Schilling	128
Meat Marinade	
Durkee 1 cup	93
French's	82
Sloppy Joe	
Ann Page	128
Durkee	118

Pizza	99
French's	128
Lawry's	139
McCormick	167
Schilling	172
Rice, Fried	
Durkee	62
Rice, Spanish	
Durkee	129
Lawry's	125
Swiss Steak	
McCormick	44
Schilling	42
Taco	
Durkee	67
French's	150
McCormick	65
Schilling	65
Tuna Casserole	
McCormick	104

DIPS, 1 oz

Ready to Serve

Bacon and Horseradish	
Borden	79
Kraft	
Ready	71
Teez	57
Lucerne	63
Bacon and Smoke	
Sealtest	47
Barbecue	
Borden's	48
Bean	
Chili	
Lucerne	50
Jalapeño	
Frito-Lay	36
Gebhardt	30
Granny Goose	37
Lucerne	35
Blue Cheese	
Granny Goose	110
Kraft	
Ready	69
Teez	51

Lucerne	67
Sealtest	49
Casino	
Sealtest	45
Chili, Green	
Borden	55
Chipped Beef	
Sealtest	44
Clam	
Kraft	
Ready	66
Teez	44
Lucerne	34
Clam and Lobster	
Borden	60
Dill	
Kraft	67
Garlic	
Granny Goose	100
Kraft	47
Lucerne	58
Green Goddess	
Kraft	45
Guacamole	
Lucerne	69
Hickory Smoke	
Lucerne	60
Onion	
Borden	48
Lawry's	50

Kraft	
Ready	68
Teez	43
Lucerne	58
Sealtest	46
Tartar	
Borden	48

Unprepared Mixes

Bacon and Onion	
Frito-Lay	100
Barbecue	
Salada	120
Blue Cheese	
Frito-Lay	117
Lawry's	94
Caesar	
Frito-Lay	118
Lawry's	94
Cheddar Cheese	
Salada	43
Chili	
Frito-Lay	120
Dill	
Frito-Lay	90
Dill and Chives	
Salada	130

Garlic and Onion	
McCormick	126
Salada	100
Horseradish	
Lawry's	86
Frito-Lay	105
Onion	
Frito-Lay	87
Green	100
Lawry's	
Green	100
Toasted	82
McCormick	131
Salada	100
Taco	
Frito-Lay	105

SALAD DRESSINGS,
1 Tbsp unless noted

Avocado	
Kraft	70
Bacon	
Lawry's	78
Blue Cheese	
Ann Page Low Calorie	18

Kraft	
Chunky	70
Low Calorie	14
Low Calorie Chunky	30
Lawry's	
bottled	57
mix, 1 pkg	74
Nu Made	75
Roka	60
Seven Seas	70
Wish-Bone	80
Weight Watchers	10
Caesar	
Kraft	70
Lawry's	
bottled	70
mix, 1 pkg	72
Nu Made	75
Pfeiffer	70
Low Calorie	10
Seven Seas	70
Wish-Bone	80
Chef Style	
Ann Page	20
Kraft	18
Coach House	
Seven Seas	78
Coleslaw	
Kraft	70
Low Calorie	30

Cucumber	
Kraft	80
Low Calorie	30
French	
Ann Page	25
Casino	70
Kraft	60
Casino Garlic	70
Herb and Garlic	90
Low Calorie	25
Miracle	70
Lawry's	
bottled	50
mix, 1 pkg	72
Nu Made	
Low Calorie	20
Savory	65
Zesty	70
Pfeiffer	55
Low Calorie	18
Seven Seas	60
Low Calorie	30
Tillie Lewis	12
Wish-Bone	
Deluxe	50
French Garlic	70
Low Calorie	25
Sweet and Spicy	70
Weight Watchers	4

Garlic	
Kraft	50
Wish-Bone	80
Green Goddess	
Kraft	80
Lawry's	
bottled	60
mix, 1 pkg	69
Nu Made	80
Seven Seas	80
Wish-Bone	60
Green Onion	
Kraft	70
Hawaiian	
Lawry's	75
Herb and Garlic	
Kraft	83
Herb and Spices	
Seven Seas	60
Italian	
Ann Page	14
Good Seasons	8
Kraft	80
Golden	70
Low Calorie	6
Lawry's	
bottled	80
mix, 1 pkg	44
cheeses mix, 1 pkg	69

Nu Made	90
Low Calorie	16
Pfeiffer	60
Low Calorie	10
Seven Seas	70
Family	60
Low Calorie	35
Viva	70
Tillie Lewis	6
Weight Watchers	2
Wish-Bone	80
Low Calorie	20
Lemon garlic	
Lawry's, 1 pkg	65
Mayonnaise, all brands	100
Mayonnaise, flavored	
Durkee	69
Mayonnaise, imitation	
Mrs. Filbert's	40
Piedmont	50
Weight Watchers	40
May Lo Naise	
Tillie Lewis	25
Oil and Vinegar	
Kraft	70
Lawry's	55
Nu Made	60
Seven Seasons	70
Onion	
Lawry's	84

Wish-Bone	80
Parmesan	
Good Seasons	84
Roquefort	
Kraft	58
Red Wine	
Pfeiffer	40
Low Calorie	10
Russian	
Kraft	30
Nu Made	55
Pfeiffer	65
Low Calorie	15
Seven Seas	80
Tillie Lewis	12
Weight Watchers	
bottled	50
mix	4
Wish-Bone	60
Low Calorie	25
Salad dressing	
Ann Page	70
Heinz	63
Kraft	65
Mrs. Filbert's	65
Nu Made	80
Piedmont	70
Sultana	50
Salad Secret	
Kraft	60

Sea Island	
Kraft	93
Sour Treat	
Friendship	90
Sherry	
Lawry's	55
Spin Blend	
Hellmann's	55
Tahitian Isle	
Wish-Bone	55
Thousand Island	
Ann Page	25
Kraft	60
Low Calorie	30
Lawry's	
bottled	65
mix, 1 pkg	78
Nu Made	30
Pfeiffer	65
Low Calorie	15
Seven Seas	50
Tillie Lewis	18
Weight Watchers	
bottled	50
mix	12
Wish-Bone	70
Low Calorie	25
Tomato-Blue Cheese	
Kraft	90

Tomato-Spice	
Seven Seas	45
Whipped	
Tillie Lewis	25
Yogonaise	
Henri's	60
Yogowhip	
Henri's	60
Yogurt, all flavors	
Henri's	35

OILS, 1 Tbsp

Corn	
Mazola	122
Nu Made	124
Olive	
Filippo Berio	125
Peanut	
Planters	128
Popcorn	
Planters	130
Safflower	
Nu Made	119
Soybean	
Mrs. Tucker's	128

Sunflower	
Sunlight	120
Vegetable	
Crisco	120
Puritan	118
Swift	115
Wesson	120
Vegetable and cottonseed	
Swift	120

Shortening, 1 Tbsp unless noted

Lard	115
1 cup	1,850
Vegetable	
Crisco	109
Fluffo	109
Mrs. Tucker's	120
Pam	7
Snowdrift	111
Spry	97

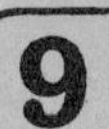

SAUCES,
½ cup unless noted

A la King	
Durkee	66
Barbecue, 1 Tbsp	
Chris' and Pitt's	15
Durkee with vinegar	64
French's	14
Hot	27
Smoky	14
Open Pit	26
Hot 'n Spicy	27
Hickory Smoked	27
with onions	28
Bearnaise	
Butternut Farm	176
Bordelaise	
Butternut Farm	48
Cheese	
Durkee	168
French's	160
McCormick	156
Schilling	156
Chili	
Gebhardt	156
Heinz	17

Hunt's	18
McCormick	92
Clam	
Buitoni	
red	102
white	114
La Rosa	
red	78
white	68
Cocktail Sauce	
Crosse & Blackwell	26
Tastee	25
Enchilada	
Gebhardt	68
Lawry's, 1 pkg	144
McCormick, 1 pkg	116
Old El Paso	
Hot	36
Mild	40
Hollandaise	
Durkee	118
French's	119
McCormick	171
Schilling	170
Horseradish, 1 oz	
Kraft	100
Italian	
Contadina	85
Lawry's, 1 pkg	86
Ragu	36

Lemon-Butter, 1 oz	
Weight Watchers	16
Mint Sauce, 1 tsp	
Crosse & Blackwell	16
Mushroom, 1 oz	
Dawn Fresh	9
Pizza	
Buitoni	92
Ragu	96
Seafood cocktail sauce, 1 tsp	
Del Monte	18
Pfeiffer	25
Sour Cream	
Durkee	160
French's	280
McCormick	146
Schilling	146
Soy Sauce, 1 tsp	
La Choy	7
Spaghetti	
Ann Page	70
Marinara	70
Meat	80
Mix, 1 envelope	120
with Mushrooms	70
Buitoni	92
Clam, red	108
Clam, white	144
Marinara	88
Meat	120

with Mushrooms	88
Durkee	45
with Mushrooms	40
French's	80
with Mushrooms	80
Franco-American	95
with Mushrooms	95
Lawry's	147
with Meatball seasoning	316
with Mushrooms	116
La Rosa	74
Prince	90
with Meat	143
with Mushrooms	103
Ragu	
Plain	96
Thick	84
Clam	88
Marinara	96
Meat	92
Thick with Meatball seasoning	104
with Mushrooms	84
Spatini	51
Town House	80
with Meat	80
with Mushrooms	89
Stroganoff	
Durkee	410
French's	165
Lawry's, 1 pkg	118

McCormick	115
Schilling	115
Sweet and Sour	
Contadina	158
Durkee	115
French's	55
La Choy	262
Swiss Steak	
Contadina	48
Taco Sauce	
Gebhardt	3
Old El Paso	4
Tartar Sauce	
Best Foods	70
Hellman's	75
Kraft	72
Lawry's	67
Seven Seas	80
Teriyaki, 1 Tbsp	
Chun King	12
French's	17
Tomato	
Contadina	45
Del Monte	40
with Bits	40
with Mushrooms	50
with Onions	50
Hunt's	35
Prima Salsa	109
Prima Salsa with Mushrooms	110

Special	40
with Bits	35
with Cheese	71
with Herbs	80
with Meat	120
with Mushrooms	40
with Onions	45
Stokely-Van Camp	35
Town House	40
Tomato Paste	
Contadina	46
Hunt's	108
Lord Mott	44
Tuna Casserole	
McCormick	128
Schilling	128
White	
Durkee	119
Wine, 1 oz	
Lawry's	
Burgundy	98
Sherry	94
White	113
Worcestershire Sauce	
Crosse & Blackwell	15
Heinz	11
French's	10
Lea & Perrins	12

Gravies, ¼ cup unless noted

Au Jus	
Ann Page 1 envelope	64
Durkee	8
Durkee, Roastin' Bag, 1 pkg	64
French's	8
French's Pan Rich	30
McCormick	4
Schilling	4
Beef	
Franco-American	30
Howard Johnson's	25
Wyler's	24
Brown	
Ann Page 1 envelope	79
Dawn Fresh	20
Durkee	15
with Mushrooms	15
with Onions	17
Franco-American	25
French's	20
French's Pan Rich	62
McCormick	26
Herb	21
Lite	10
Pillsbury	15
Schilling	26
Herb	21

Weight Watchers	8
with Mushrooms	12
with Onions	13
Chicken	
Ann Page, 1 envelope	120
College Inn	25
Durkee	22
Creamy	39
Roastin' Bag, 1 pkg	122
Roastin' Bag Italian, 1 pkg	144
French's	25
French's Pan Rich	60
McCormick	21
Lite	10
Pillsbury	25
Schilling	21
Lite	10
Weight Watchers	10
Wyler's	24
Chicken Giblet	
Franco-American	35
Herb	
McCormick	26
Homestyle	
Durkee	18
French's	25
Pillsbury	15
Meatloaf	
Durkee, 1 pkg	130

Mushroom	
Ann Page, 1 envelope	79
Durkee	16
Franco-American	35
French's	20
McCormick	19
Schilling	19
Wyler's	15
Mustard	
French's	16
Onion	
Ann Page, 1 envelope	120
Durkee	21
Durkee Roastin' Bag, 1 pkg	124
French's	25
French's Pan Rich	50
Pork	
Durkee	18
Durkee Roastin' Bag, 1 pkg	130
French's	20
Pot Roast	
Durkee, 1 pkg	124
Sparerib	
Durkee, 1 pkg	162
Swiss Steak	
Durkee	11
Durkee Roastin' Bag, 1 pkg	115
Turkey	
Durkee	23

French's	25
McCormick	21
Schilling	22
Turkey Giblet	
Howard Johnson's	28

CHAPTER 10

Desserts, Baking and Baked Goods

BAKING MISCELLANY

Baking Powder, 1 tsp	5
Yeast, ¼ oz unless noted	
Baker's	6
Brewer's	20
Dry, active	
Fleischmann's	20
Fresh, active	
Fleischmann's .6 oz pkg	15
Household	
Fleischmann's	7
Torula	20

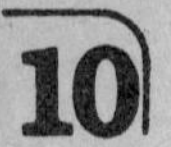

Baking Chocolate, 1 oz	
Chips	
Baker's	130
Hershey's	115
Nestlé	130
Ground	
Ghiradelli	150
Solid	
Baker's	
German	140
semi-sweet	130
unsweetened	140
Ghiradelli	150
Hershey	190
Butterscotch	
Nestlé chips	150
Coconut	
Baker's	150
Ginger	
Borden's crystallized	98
Borden's preserved	88
Peanut Butter	
Reese chips	150

CAKES, FROZEN,
1 whole cake

Banana	
Pepperidge Farm	1,115
Sara Lee	1,439
Banana Nut	
Sara Lee	1,864
Black Forest	
Sara Lee	1,625
Boston Creme	
Pepperidge Farm	1,070
Cheesecake	
Lambrecht	1,530
Mrs. Smith's	1,230
Sara Lee	
small	860
large	1,440
Cherry	1,280
French	2,190
Strawberry	1,280
Strawberry French	2,062
Chocolate	
Pepperidge Farm	1,238
Sara Lee	1,380
Chocolate Bavarian	
Sara Lee	2,250

Chocolate Fudge	
Pepperidge Farm	1,800
Chocolate, German	
Pepperidge Farm	1,589
Sara Lee	1,234
Coconut	
Pepperidge Farm	1,800
Crumbcake	
Sara Lee	170
Stouffer's	
Blueberry	211
Chocolate Chip	225
French	200
Cupcake	
Stouffer's	
Cream	240
Yellow	190
Devil's Food	
Pepperidge Farm	1,800
Sara Lee	1,496
Golden	
Pepperidge Farm	900
Sara Lee	1,440
Lemon	
Sara Lee	2,175
Lemon Coconut	
Pepperidge Farm	1,100
Mandarin Orange	
Sara Lee	1,650

Orange	
Howard Johnson's	1,700
Sara Lee	1,440
Pound	
Sara Lee	
Banana Nut	1,170
Chocolate	1,220
Chocolate Swirl	1,300
Plain	1,320
Raisin	1,270
Pepperidge Farm	
Apple Nut	1,300
Butter	1,300
Carrot	1,600
Chocolate	1,300
Cherry	
Mrs. Smith's	2,335
Strawberry	
Mrs. Smith's	1,830
Sara Lee	1,550
Strawberry and Cream	1,700
Vanilla	
Pepperidge Farm	1,900
Walnut	
Sara Lee	1,690

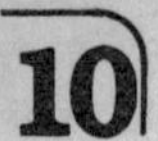

CAKE MIXES, 1 whole cake

Angel Food	
Betty Crocker	1,560
One Step	1,680
Confetti	1,800
Strawberry	1,800
Duncan Hines	1,670
Pillsbury	1,680
Swans Down	1,590
Apple Raisin	
Duncan Hines	2,280
Spicy	1,620
Applesauce Raisin	
Betty Crocker	1,800
Banana	
Betty Crocker	3,140
Duncan Hines	2,400
Pillsbury	3,120
Banana Nut	
Betty Crocker	1,800
Duncan Hines	1,800
Bundt	
Pillsbury	
Fudge	3,480
Lemon	3,350
Macaroon	3,950
Marble	3,960

Pound	3,710
Triple Fudge	3,590
Butter	
Duncan Hines	3,240
Pillsbury	2,680
Butter Brickle	
Betty Crocker	3,110
Butter Fudge	
Duncan Hines	3,240
Butter Pecan	
Betty Crocker	3,120
Cheesecake	
Jello-O	2,000
Pillsbury	3,120
Royal	1,840
Cherry	
Duncan Hines	2,280
Cherry Chip	
Betty Crocker	2,280
Chocolate	
Betty Crocker	1,380
Duncan Hines	2,400
Pillsbury Dark	3,120
Swans Down	2,240
Chocolate Almond	
Betty Crocker	1,890
Chocolate Chip	
Betty Crocker	1,980
Duncan Hines	1,710
Double Chocolate Chip	1,620

Chocolate Fudge	
Betty Crocker	3,240
Chocolate, German	
Betty Crocker	3,240
Pillsbury	3,120
Chocolate, Sour Cream	
Betty Crocker	3,240
Duncan Hines	2,400
Chocolate, Swiss	
Duncan Hines	2,400
Swans Down	2,240
Chocolate with frosting	
Betty Crocker	1,620
Coconut Pecan	
Betty Crocker	1,975
Date Nut	
Betty Crocker	1,890
Devil's Food	
Betty Crocker	3,240
Duncan Hines	2,400
Pillsbury	3,240
Swans Down	2,230
Fudge Marble	
Duncan Hines	2,400
Pillsbury	3,240
Gingerbread	
Betty Crocker	1,890
Lemon	
Betty Crocker	3,240
Pudding Cake	1,380

Duncan Hines	2,400
Pillsbury	3,240
Lemon Chiffon	
Betty Crocker	2,280
Marble	
Betty Crocker	3,280
Orange	
Betty Crocker	3,240
Duncan Hines	2,400
Pineapple	
Betty Crocker	2,400
Duncan Hines	2,400
Pound	
Betty Crocker	2,280
Spice	
Betty Crocker	3,240
Duncan Hines	2,400
Spice Raisin	
Betty Crocker	1,800
Strawberry	
Betty Crocker	3,240
Duncan Hines	2,400
Streusel	
Pillsbury	
Cinnamon	4,080
Devil's Food	3,950
Fudge Marble	4,080
Chocolate	3,950
Lemon	4,200

White	
Betty Crocker	2,400
Duncan Hines	2,280
Pillsbury	3,000
Swans Down	2,120
Yellow	
Betty Crocker	3,240
Butter	2,880
with frosting	1,380
Duncan Hines	2,400
Pillsbury	3,120
Swans Down	2,240

CAKES FOR SNACKS, 1 cake

Big Wheels	170
Brownie	
Hostess	
small	150
large	240
Chocolate, cream-filled	
Yankee Doodles	134
Choco-Diles	250
Creamies, 1 pkg	
Tastykake	
Chocolate	255

Spice	270
Crumb Cakes	
Hostess	130
Cupcakes	
Hostess	
Chocolate	155
Orange	147
Tastykake, 1 pkg	
Buttercream	238
Chocolate	200
Chocolate Cream	239
Devil Dogs	169
Devil's Food	
Hostess	140
Drake's	135
Ding Dongs	170
Donuts	
Hostess	
Cinnamon	110
Crunch	100
Enrobed	130
Plain	105
Powdered	115
Funny Bones, 1 pkg	162
Ho-Ho's	120
Juniors, 1 pkg	
Tastykake	
Chocolate	307
Coconut	330
Coffee cake	310

Krimpets, 1 pkg	
Tastykake	
Butterscotch	190
Chocolate	255
Jelly	168
Vanilla	240
Macaroons	
Hostess	210
Oatmeal Raisin, 1 pkg	
Tastykake	267
Orange Treats, 1 pkg	
Tastykake	230
Pound	
Drake's	
Marble	185
Plain	181
Raisin	323
Ring Ding	366
Sno Balls	140
Tandy Takes, 1 pkg	
Chocolate	180
Peanut Butter	190
Teens, 1 pkg	225
Tempty, 1 pkg	
Chocolate	196
Lemon	259
Tiger Tails	415
Twinkies	140

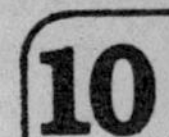

COFFEE CAKE, 1 cake

Almond	
Sara Lee	1,350
Sara Lee Coffee Ring	1,100
Angel Food	
Howard Johnson's	710
Apple	
Morton	1,130
Sara Lee	1,175
Apple Cinnamon	
Pillsbury	1,880
Apricot	
Sara Lee	1,176
Banana	
Sara Lee	1,440
Blueberry	
Sara Lee Coffee Ring	1,080
Sara Lee Danish	1,175
Butter Pecan	
Pillsbury	2,480
Butter Streusel	
Sara Lee	1,395
Cherry	
Sara Lee	1,050
Chocolate	
Sara Lee	1,375

Chocolate, German	
Morton	1,360
Sara Lee	1,230
Cinnamon Streusel	
Pillsbury	2,000
Sara Lee	1,230
Coconut	
Pepperidge Farm	1,940
Coffee Cake	
Aunt Jemima	1,360
Crumb	
Drake's	1,460
Lemon	
Drake's	1,030
Maple Crunch	
Sara Lee	1,157
Orange	
Sara Lee	1,442
Pecan	
Drake's	1,109
Morton	1,368
Sara Lee small	764
Sara Lee large	1,320
Raspberry	
Sara Lee	1,090
Sour Cream	
Pillsbury	2,160

COOKIES, 1 piece

Adelaide	
Pepperidge Farm	53
Almond	
Keebler	47
Stella D'Oro	49
Almond Spice	
Keebler	50
Angel Puffs	
Stella D'Oro	17
Animal Crackers	
Keebler	12
Nabisco	12
Sunshine	10
Animal Crackers Iced	
Keebler	52
Sunshine	26
Anise	
Stella D'Oro	
Anisette Sponge	50
Anisette Toast	34
Apple	
Keebler	27
Nabisco	48
Applesauce	
Sunshine	33
Iced	104

Arrowroot	
Nabisco	22
Sunshine	16
Assorted	
Stella D'Oro	
Hostess	39
Lady Stella	37
Bordeaux	
Pepperidge Farm	37
Breakfast Treats	
Stella D'Oro	100
Brown Edge	
Nabisco	28
Brown Sugar	
Nabisco	25
Pepperidge Farm	50
Brussels	
Pepperidge Farm	57
Butter	
Keebler	84
Nabisco	37
Pepperidge Farm	38
Sunshine	24
Capri	
Pepperidge Farm	85
Cashew	
Nabisco	57
Chessman	
Pepperidge Farm	43

Chinese Dessert	
Stella D'Oro	170
Chocolate	
Keebler	
Bavarian Fudge	80
Nut Fudge	31
Pecan Fudge	66
Melody	31
Nabisco	
Wafers	28
Snaps	18
Pepperidge Farm	48
Sunshine	13
Chocolate Almond	
Nabisco	55
Chocolate Brownies	
Pepperidge Farm	57
Chocolate Chip	
Chips Ahoy	50
Estee	30
Keebler	44
Old Fashioned	80
Rich 'N Chips	73
Townhouse	49
Nabisco	51
Family Favorite	33
Snaps	21
Pepperidge Farm	52
Sunshine	37
Chip-A-Roos	63

Chocolate Chip Coconut	
Keebler	80
Nabisco	76
Sunshine	76
Chocolate Strawberry Wafers	
Estee	90
Cinnamon	
Sunshine	20
Cinnamon Almond	
Nabisco	53
Cinnamon Sugar	
Fun Days	48
Pepperidge Farm	52
Coconut	
Keebler	61
Old Fashioned	83
Strip	37
Nabisco	16
Stella D'Oro	47
Sunshine	47
Coconut, Iced	
Keebler Crunchies	70
Coconut Chocolate	
Pepperidge Farm	83
Creme Sandwiches	
Butterscotch	
Keebler	85
Chocolate	
Keebler Dutch	95

Keebler Opera	85
Oreo grocery	50
Oreo individual	40
Chocolate fudge	
Cookie Mates	53
Keebler	97
Sunshine	74
Coconut	
Nabisco	53
Sunshine	51
Wise Coco	39
Lemon	
Keebler	85
Swiss	
Nabisco	43
Vanilla	
Cameo	68
Cookie Mates	52
Keebler	82
French	95
Opera	85
Sunshine	79
Vienna Fingers	69
Wise	38
Crescents	
Nabisco	34
Cup Custard	
Sunshine	70
Danish Wedding	
Keebler	31

Date Nut	
Pepperidge Farm	53
Sunshine	82
Devil's Food	
Keebler	64
Nabisco	58
Sunshine	55
Dixie Vanilla	
Sunshine	60
Egg Biscuits	
Stella D'Oro	37
Anise	135
Egg Jumbo	43
Rum and Brandy	135
Sugared	135
Vanilla	130
Figs	
Nabisco Fig Newtons	59
Frito-Lay	189
Keebler	71
Sunshine	42
Fruit	
Stella D'Oro	67
Sunshine Golden Fruit	61
Fruit, Iced	
Nabisco	70
Fudge	
Keebler	
Sticks	42

Strips	57
Pepperidge Farm	58
Gingerbread	
Pepperidge Farm	33
Gingerbread, Iced	
Keebler	130
Ginger Snaps	
Keebler	39
Nabisco	30
Sunshine	
small	14
large	32
Golden Bars	
Stella D'Oro	110
Graham Crackers	
Keebler	
Honey	17
Thin	17
Very Thin	14
Nabisco	30
Honey Maid	30
Sunshine	17
Sugar Honey	30
Graham Crackers, chocolate covered	
Keebler	44
Milco	91
Nabisco	55
Fancy Dip	68
Pantry	62
Robena	72

Kichel	
Stella D'Oro	64
Lady Joan	
Sunshine	42
Sunshine Iced	47
LaLanne	
Sunshine	15
Lemon	
Keebler	83
Nabisco	17
Sunshine	76
Lemon Coolers	29
Lemon Nut	
Pepperidge Farm	58
Lido	
Pepperidge Farm	95
Love Cookies	
Stella D'Oro	110
Macaroons	
Sunshine	85
Butter	39
Coconut	81
Bake Shop	87
Nabisco	71
Mandel Toast	
Stella D'Oro	54
Margherite	
Stella D'Oro	73
Marigold Sandwich	
Keebler	9

Marshmallow

Chocolate covered	
Keebler	
Dainties	68
Galaxies	82
Treasures	83
Tulips	83
Coconut	
Nabisco	54
Sunshine	70
Iced	
Sunshine	
Frosted Cakes	68
Nut Sundae	74
Mallomars	60
Nabisco	
Puffs	94
Twirls	133
Pinwheels	139
Sunshine	
Puffs	63
Kings	135
Sandwich	
Keebler	81
Nabisco	32
Sprinkles	
Sunshine	71

Milano

Pepperidge Farm	63
Mint	70

Molasses Crisps	
Pepperidge Farm	30
Molasses and Spice	
Sunshine	67
Nassau	
Pepperidge Farm	75
Oatmeal	
Keebler	78
Nabisco	
Family Favorite	24
Home Style	60
Sunshine	63
Oatmeal Almond	
Pepperidge Farm	53
Oatmeal, Iced	
Keebler	82
Oatmeal Marmalade	
Pepperidge Farm	53
Oatmeal Peanut Butter	
Sunshine	79
Oatmeal Raisin	
Bake Shop	76
Nabisco	77
Pepperidge Farm	54
Orleans	
Pepperidge Farm	3[illegible]
Peanut	
Pepperidge Farm	4[illegible]
Sunshine	3[illegible]

Peanut Butter	
Keebler	81
Nabisco Nutter Butter	69
Sunshine	
Crunch	68
Patties	30
Peanut Butter, Chocolate-covered	
Eton	53
Keebler	117
Peanut Caramel	
Hey Days	122
Peanut Cream	
Nabisco	34
Pecan	
Keebler	20
Sunshine	78
Pfeffernusse	
Stella D'Oro	44
Pirouette	
Pepperidge Farm	40
Prune	
Stella D'Oro	87
Raisin	
Nabisco	56
Stella D'Oro	115
Sunshine	73
Raisin, Iced	
Keebler	81

Raisin Bran	
Pepperidge Farm	53
Shortbread	
Keebler	27
Lorna Doone	38
Pepperidge Farm	65
Scottie	39
Shortbread with Cashews	
Nabisco	50
Shortbread, Chocolate-covered	
Nabisco	50
Shortbread with Coconut	65
Shortbread, Iced	58
Shortbread Pecans	
Keebler	77
Nabisco	77
St. Moritz	
Pepperidge Farm	47
Sorrento	
Stella D'Oro	57
Sprinkles	
Sunshine	57
Sugar	
Eton	50
Keebler	
Giant	70
Old Fashioned	81
Nabisco	17
Pepperidge Farm	53

Sugar Wafers	
Nabisco Biscos	18
Creme Waffles	47
Keebler	26
Kreemlined	45
Regent	23
Sunshine	47
Sugar Wafers, Chocolate-covered	
Eton	54
Milco	80
Nabisco	76
Creme Stix	50
Sunshine	30
Sugar Wafers, Spiced	
Nabisco	33
Sunflower Raisin	
Pepperidge Farm	53
Swedish Creme	103
Swiss Chalet	97
Swiss Fudge	
Stella D'Oro	64
Tahiti	
Pepperidge Farm	85
Taste of Vienna	
Stella D'Oro	85
Tea Biscuits	
Nabisco	21
Toy Cookies	
Sunshine	13

Vanilla	
Keebler	19
Nabisco	
Snaps	13
Wafers	18
Sunshine	15
Vanilla Thins	
Estee	25
Vienna Finger Sandwich	
Sunshine	71
Yum Yums	
Sunshine	83
Zanzibar	
Pepperidge Farm	37

PASTRY, FROZEN, MIXES, AND TOASTER, 1 piece unless noted

Dessert mixes	
Pillsbury Appleasy	160
Donuts	
Morton	
Bavarian Creme	180
Boston Creme	205

Chocolate	150
Glazed	150
Jelly	180
Mini	120
Town House Cinnamon	210
Dumplings, apple	
Pepperidge Farm	280
Strudel, apple	
Pepperidge Farm, 1 oz	85
Tarts	
Kellogg's Pop Tarts	210
Pepperidge Farm	
Apple	280
Blueberry	285
Cherry	280
Lemon	310
Raspberry	320
Popovers (Flako)	166
Turnovers	
Pepperidge Farm	320
Pillsbury	180

PIES, FROZEN, 1 whole pie

Apple	
Banquet	1,440

Morton	1,740
Mini	590
Mrs. Smith's	1,768
Natural	2,881
Dutch	1,860
Tart	1,495
Banana Cream	
Banquet	1,032
Morton	1,020
Mini	230
Mrs. Smith's	1,290
Light	1,320
Blueberry	
Banquet	1,523
Morton	1,680
Mini	580
Mrs. Smith's	1,740
Natural	2,040
Boston Cream	
Mrs. Smith's	1,980
Cherry	
Banquet	1,360
Morton	1,805
Mini	591
Mrs. Smith's	1,860
Natural	2,040
Chocolate	
Mrs. Smith's	1,500
Royal Dutch	2,040

Chocolate Cream	
Banquet	1,060
Morton	1,200
Mini	260
Mrs. Smith's	1,470
Coconut	
Mrs. Smith's	1,380
Coconut Cream	
Banquet	1,040
Morton	1,140
Mini	260
Mrs. Smith's	1,380
Coconut Custard	
Banquet	1,220
Morton	
Mini	370
Mrs. Smith's	1,590
Custard	
Banquet	1,240
Devil Cream	
Royal	2,280
Mrs. Smith's	1,470
Lemon	
Mrs. Smith's	2,040
Royal	2,080
Lemon Cream	
Banquet	1,000
Morton	1,000
Mini	240
Mrs. Smith's	1,350

Lemon Crunch	
Mrs. Smith's	2,480
Lemon Meringue	
Mrs. Smith's	1,560
Lemon Yogurt	
Mrs. Smith's	1,200
Mince	
Morton	1,860
Mini	590
Mrs. Smith's	2,010
Mincemeat	
Banquet	1,520
Neapolitan Cream	
Morton	1,140
Mrs. Smith's	1,440
Nesselrode	
Royal	2,000
Peach	
Banquet	1,320
Morton	1,680
Mini	560
Mrs. Smith's	1,800
Natural	1,980
Pecan	
Morton	
Mini	580
Mrs. Smith's	2,589
Pineapple	
Mrs. Smith's	1,800

Pineapple-Cheese	
Mrs. Smith's	1,580
Pumpkin	
Banquet	1,230
Morton	1,380
Mini	430
Mrs. Smith's	1,440
Raisin	
Mrs. Smith's	1,890
Spumoni	
Royal	2,120
Strawberry Cream	
Banquet	1,020
Morton	1,080
Mrs. Smith's	1,320
Strawberry and Rhubarb	
Mrs. Smith's	1,890
Natural	1,920
Strawberry-Yogurt	
Mrs. Smith's	1,220

Pie Mixes, 1 whole pie

Betty Crocker Boston Cream	2,080
Pillsbury	
Chocolate Cream	2,460
Lemon Chiffon	1,980
Vanilla	2,340

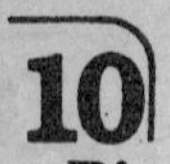

Pie Crusts and Shells, 1 piece

Pastry Sheets	
Pepperidge Farm	570
Pastry Shells	
Pepperidge Farm	240
Stella D'Oro	146
Pie Crusts	
Betty Crocker	1,920
Stick	960
Flako	1,560
Pillsbury	1,740
Pie Shells	
Pepperidge Farm	521
shallow	440
with top	760
Stella D'Oro	240
Tart Shells	
Pepperidge Farm	88

Pie Fillings, 1 whole can unless noted

Apple	
Wilderness	660
Apricot	
Wilderness	720
Banana Cream	
Jell-O	660

Blueberry	
Wilderness	660
Cherry	
Wilderness	650
Lemon	
Jell-O	1,080
Royal, 1 cup	310
Wilderness	840
Lime	
Royal, 1 cup	310
Mince	
Wilderness	840
Mincemeat	
None Such, 1 cup	660
Peach	
Wilderness	655
Pumpkin	
Libby's, 1 cup	205
Stokely-Van Camp, 1 cup	370
Raisin	
Wilderness	720
Strawberry	
Wilderness	710

SMALL PASTRY PIES, 1 piece

Apple	
Stella D'Oro	90
Hostess	400
Tastykake	350
Tastykake French	400
Blueberry	
Hostess	365
Cherry	
Hostess	420
Tastykake	380
Fig	
Stella D'Oro	100
Guava	
Stella D'Oro	125
Lemon	
Hostess	420
Tastykake	355
Peach/Apricot	
Stella D'Oro	90
Pecan	
Frito-Lay	345
Prune	
Stella D'Oro	92
Puff Pastry	
Durkee	
Beef	47

Cheese	59
Chicken	49
Chicken liver	48
Shrimp	44

PUDDINGS, MIXES AND CANNED, ½ cup, unless noted

Banana	
Ann Page	250
Del Monte	180
Shak-A-Pudd'n	165
Royal	164
Banana Cream	
Jell-O	175
My-T-Fine	175
Bavarian Cream	
My-T-Fine	176
Butter Pecan	
My-T-Fine	175
Butterscotch	
Ann Page	190
Instant	170
Del Monte	175

D-Zerta	25
Foremost	175
Jell-O	172
My-T-Fine	170
Royal	190
Sego	250
Caramel Nut	
Royal	195
Cherry	
Whip 'n Chill	139
Cherry-Plum	
Junket	135
Chocolate	
Ann Page	180
Betty Crocker	180
Bounty	174
Dannon	150
Del Monte	250
D-Zerta	20
Foremost	175
Jell-O	175
Instant	190
My-T-Fine	185
Royal	190
Dark 'N Sweet	200
Sego	250
Shak-A-Pudd'n	200
Whip 'n Chill	145
Chocolate Almond	
My-T-Fine	196

Chocolate Fudge	
Betty Crocker	180
Del Monte	190
Foremost	175
Jell-O	175
Instant	191
My-T-Fine	190
Sego	250
Whip 'n Chill	139
Chocolate Malt	
Shak-A-Pudd'n	200
Chocolate Marshmallow	
Sego	250
Coconut	
Ann Page	
Cream	190
Toasted	170
Jell-O	175
Instant	190
Royal	185
Currant-Raspberry	
Junket	135
Custard	
Ann Page	150
Jell-O	165
My-T-Fine	
Caramel	145
Vanilla	156
Rice-A-Roni	120
Royal	145

Indian	
B & M	150
Lemon	
Ann Page	150
Instant	180
Bounty	196
Foremost	197
Jell-O	178
Instant	179
My-T-Fine	180
Royal	180
Whip 'n Chill	135
Lemon Chiffon	
Jell-O	144
Mocha Nut	
Royal	190
Pineapple Cream	
Jell-O	165
Instant	179
Pistachio	
Ann Page	180
Royal	180
Plum	
Crosse & Blackwell	255
R & R	300
Rice	
Betty Crocker	150
Bounty	195
Strawberry	
Junket	135

Shak-A-Pudd'n	160
Whip 'n Chill	135
Tapioca	
Chocolate	
Ann Page	180
Jell-O	165
Royal	185
Lemon	
Jell-O	166
Orange	
Jell-O	166
Vanilla	
Ann Page	170
Betty Crocker	150
Jell-O	166
My-T-Fine	144
Royal	170
Vanilla	
Ann Page	170
Betty Crocker	190
Bounty	128
Dannon	150
Del Monte	190
D-Zerta	30
Foremost	175
Jell-O	164
Instant	178
My-T-Fine	170
Royal	165
Instant	180

Sego	250
Shak-A-Pudd'n	165
Whip 'n Chill	135

CHAPTER 11

Jellies, Syrups, Toppings and Spreads

DESSERT TOPPINGS, 1 Tbsp

Black Cherry	
No-Cal	0
Black Raspberry	
No-Cal	0
Butterscotch	
Hershey's	55
Kraft	60
Smucker's	69
Caramel	
Kraft	
chocolate	56

vanilla	57
Smucker's	69
peanut butter	75
Cherry	
Smucker's	65
Chocolate	
Bosco	50
Hershey's	45
Kraft	50
No-Cal	6
Smucker's	65
Tillie Lewis	16
Chocolate Fudge	
Hershey's	45
Kraft	70
Smucker's	65
Swiss	72
Chocolate Mint	
Hershey's	61
Smucker's	67
Chocolate Peanut Butter	
Hershey's	60
Coffee	
No-Cal	6
Cola	
No-Cal	0
Cream, whipped	
Reddi-Whip	8
Top-Whip	7

Grape	
No-Cal	0
Hard Sauce	
Crosse & Blackwell	64
Marshmallow	
Kraft	35
Pecans in Syrup	
Kraft	82
Smucker's	65
Pineapple	
Kraft	50
Smucker's	62
Strawberry	
Kraft	45
No-Cal	0
Smucker's	60
Walnut	
Kraft	88
Walnuts in Syrup	
Smucker's	65
Whip, non-dairy	
Cool Whip	14
D-Zerta	8
Dream Whip	10
Kraft	9
Lucky Whip	11
Pet	16
Reddi-Whip	9

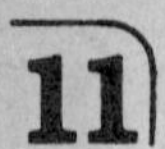

FROSTINGS, 1 can

Betty Crocker	
Chocolate Fudge	1920
Coconut Pecan	1310
White, creamy	1920
White, fluffy *Lite*	720
All other flavors	1800
Pillsbury	
Coconut Pecan	1800
White, fluffy	840
All other flavors	2040

GELATIN, ½ cup

Borden's	
Cherry	80
Fruit Cocktail	109
Mandarin Orange	89
Perfection	81
Pineapple-papaya	78
Pineapple-raspberry	77
Strawberry	75

Jell-O	
1-2-3	81
Best	77
Knox **unflavored, dry, 1 envelope**	28
Royal	80

JELLIES AND BUTTERS, 1 Tbsp

Apple Butter	
Bama	31
Smucker's	
Cider	39
Spiced	39
Peach	45
Ma Brown	32
Musselman's	33
Jams	
Ann Page	51
Bama	51
Diet Delight	22
Kraft	49
S & W	10
Smucker's	54
Slenderella	24
artificially sweetened	1

Jellies

Ann Page	54
Bama	51
Crosse & Blackwell	51
Diet Delight	21
Home Brands	54
Kraft	48
Low Calorie	22
Ma Brown	49
Musselman's	53
S & W	12
Smucker's	51
Slenderella	24
Single Service	50
Welch's	50

Marmalade

Ann Page	54
Bama	54
Kraft	54
Low Calorie	25
S & W	11
Smucker's	49
Slenderella	24

Preserves

Ann Page	54
Bama	51
Crosse & Blackwell	59
Empress	54
Home Brands	54
Kraft	48

Low Calorie	25
Regular	55
Ma Brown	51
S & W	11
Smucker's	54
Welch's	54
Spreads	
Smucker's	24
Tillie Lewis	12

SPREADS, 1 Tbsp

Anchovy Paste	
Crosse & Blackwell	20
Chicken	
Swanson	35
Underwood	32
Chicken Salad	
Carnation	31
Corned Beef	
Underwood	28
Ham	
Carnation	26
Hormel	35
Libby's	100
Underwood	48

Liverwurst	
Underwood	46
Peanut Butter	
Ann Page	105
Bama	100
and jelly	82
Datetree	93
Home Brands	100
Jif	93
Kitchen King	95
Peter Pan	94
Planters	95
Roberts	93
Skippy	95
Smucker's	95
Goober Grape	63
Sultana	101
Potted Meat	
Libby's	140
Roast Beef	
Underwood	29
Sandwich Spread	
Best Foods	60
Hellman's	58
Mrs. Filbert's	53
Nu Made	51
Oscar Mayer	33
Spam	
Hormel	40

Tuna	
Carnation	26
Turkey Salad	
Carnation	27

SUGAR, SYRUPS, SWEETENERS AND HONEY

Honey, 1 Tbsp	64
1 cup	1,031
Sugar, 1 cup	
Brown	
loosely packed	540
firmly packed	820
Maple	790
Powdered	460
sifted	385
White, granulated	770
1 Tbsp	45
Sweeteners, Sugar Substitutes	
Dia-Mel Sugar-Like, 1 gram pkt	3
Dia-Mel Sweet'n-it Liquid	0
Featherweight Sug'r Like, 1 tsp	2
Pillsbury Sprinkle Sweet, 1 tsp	2

Pillsbury Sweet 10	0
Sweet'n Low, 1 gram pkt	3½
Weight Watchers Sweet'ner, 1 gram pkt	3
Whitlock Suprose, 1 gram pkt	4
Syrup, 1 Tbsp	
Aunt Jemima	53
Cary's Diet	10
Cary's Maple	60
Diet Delight	15
Golden Griddle	50
Karo	60
Corn	58
Maple	54
Log Cabin	
Buttered	52
Country Kitchen	53
Maple	46
Maple-Honey	55
Mrs. Butterworth's	54
S & W	12
Tillie Lewis	14
Molasses	
dark	45
light	50
Sorghum	55

CHAPTER 12

Candies, Ice Cream and Nuts

CANDY, 1 oz

Baby Ruth	135
Butterfinger	130
Butter mint	
Kraft	8
Caramel	
Curtiss	113
Kraft	114
Sugar Daddy	113
Sugar Babies	113
Caramel, chocolate-coated	
Kraft	124

Milk Duds	111
Nestlé's Caramel Cream	124
Poms Poms	119
Certs	
clear	8
pressed	6
Cherry, chocolate-coated	
Welch's	115
Chewels	10
Chocolate, milk	
Ghiradelli	150
Hershey	152
Nestlé's	148
Welch's	116
Chocolate, mint	
Welch's	142
Chocolate, semi-sweet	
Eagle	142
Hershey	147
Nestlé's	141
Chocolate, candy-coated	
Hershey	133
Chocolate with fruit or nuts	
Chunky	135
Chunky Pecan	135
Ghiradelli	152
Hershey	154
Mr. Goodbar	153
Nestlé's	149

Jellied Candy	
Dots	100
Jujubes	50
Jujyfruits	94
Mason	99
Quaker City	93
Red Hot Dollars	94
Licorice	
Black Crows	101
Diamond Drops	98
Good & Plenty	99
Heide Pastilles	96
Switzer	97
Lifesavers, 1 piece	7
Malted Milk	
Walter Johnson	131
Mars	126
Marshmallows	
Campfire	100
Curtiss	97
Kraft	96
Jet Puff	125
Macaroon	110
Milky Way	119
Mints	
Kraft	105
Richardson	110
Mints, chocolate-coated	
Mason	203

Nestlé's	121
Welch's	108
Nougat	
Bit-O-Honey	116
Bit-O-Peanut Butter	118
Nougat, nuts and chocolate	
Oh Henry	131
Powerhouse	122
Nut Brittle	
Bonomo	115
Kraft	120
Chocolate-coated	130
Planters Cashew	135
Peanut	139
Nuts, chocolate-coated	
Hershey	
Almonds	143
Peanuts	140
Kraft	
Almonds	155
Brazil nuts	166
Peanuts	152
Welch's peanuts	157
Nuts and Caramel, chocolate-coated	
Choc-O-Nuts	132
Kraft	
Almond	155
Cashew	153
Peanut	151

Laddie Bar	133
Old Nick	134
Welch's	124
Peanut Butter, chocolate-coated	
Reese	148
Popcorn, caramel-coated	
Cracker Jack	132
King Korn	117
Old London	117
Wise	103
Raisins, chocolate-coated	
Kraft	115
Welch's	102
Snickers	128
Taffy	
Bonomo Turkish	104
Williamson Kisses	125
Toffee	
Kraft	112
chocolate-covered with almond	144
Tootsie Pops	149
Tootsie Roll	115
Trident Mints	8
Triple Decker	148

GUM, 1 piece

Adams	9
Beeman	10
Beech-Nut	9
Beechies	6
Black Jack	9
Bubble Yum	25
Bubblicious	24
Care Free	8
Chiclets	6
Clorets	6
Clove	5
Dentyne	5
Estee	3
Freshen-Up	9
Fruit Stripe	9
Orbit	8
Trident	5
Wrigley's	10

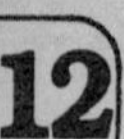

ICE CREAM, 1 cup (½ pint)

Black Raspberry	
Breyer's	264
Black Walnut	
Meadow Gold	329
Butter Almond	
Sealtest	326
Butter Almond and Chocolate	
Breyer's	318
Butter Brickle	
Sealtest	299
Butter Pecan	
Meadow Gold	300
Sealtest	322
Butterscotch Pecan	
Breyer's	302
Caramel Pecan	
Breyer's	320
Cherry	
Sealtest	276
Cherry-Vanilla	
Breyer's	280
Meadow Gold	280
Sealtest	265
Chocolate	
Borden's	255
Breyer's	314

Carnation	253
Howard Johnson's	519
Meadow Gold	278
Sealtest	281
Swift's	257
Chocolate Almond	
Breyer's	366
Dutch	299
Sealtest	324
Chocolate Chip	
Breyer's Mint	344
Meadow Gold	295
Sealtest	291
Coconut	
Sealtest	321
Coffee	
Breyer's	287
Sealtest	288
Lemon	
Sealtest	272
Maple Walnut	
Sealtest	322
Peach	
Meadow Gold	259
Sealtest	253
Pineapple	
Sealtest	251
Strawberry	
Bordens	253
Breyer's	253

Howard Johnson's	414
Meadow Gold	281
Sealtest	254
Swift's	242
Vanilla	
Bordens	246
Breyer's	299
Carnation	250
Howard Johnson's	500
Meadow Gold	280
Sealtest	289
Swift's	267
Sealtest	280
Vanilla-Fudge	
Breyer's	300
Vanilla-Raspberry	
Sealtest	279

Ice Milk, 1 cup — 200

Sherbet, 1 cup — 260

Ice Cream Bars, 1

Bi-sicle	110
Creamsicle	78
Dreamsicle	70
Dreamstick	180
Drumstick	183
Fudgesicle	100
Good Humor	
Almond	218
Chocolate	222
Ice	50
Chocolate-covered vanilla	169
Whammy	105
Popsicle	72
Sealtest	
Orange Cream	71
Orange Treat	89

Ice Cream Cones and Cups, 1 item

Comet	
cone	19
cone, rolled sugar	35
cup	20

Take-Out Ice Cream, 1 item

Baskin Robbins	
Banana Daiquiri Ice	129
Butter Pecan	195
Chocolate Fudge	229
Chocolate Mint	189
Jamoca	182
Mango Sherbert	132
Peach	165
Rocky Road	205
Strawberry	168
Vanilla	217
Bridgeman's	
Plain cone	170
Sugar cone	200
Dairy Queen	
Banana Split	540
Cone	
large	340
medium	230
small	110
Float	330
Freeze	520
Malt	
large	840
medium	600
small	340
Parfait	460
Sandwich	140

Sundae	
large	400
medium	300
small	170
Friendly's	
Fribble	
chocolate	470
vanilla	420
Sundae	
vanilla fudge	420
vanilla strawberry	340

NUTS AND SEEDS, 1 oz

Almonds	
Blue Diamond	179
Franklin	154
Granny Goose	155
Planters	170
Cashews	
A & P	170
Frito-Lay	170
Franklin	145
Granny Goose	170
Planters	170
Skippy	163

Filberts	
Franklin	164
Mixed	
A & P	190
Excel	190
Franklin	160
with peanuts	156
Granny Goose	168
Planters	180
with peanuts	185
Skippy	172
Peanuts	
A & P	180
in shell	170
Excel	180
Frito-Lay	175
in shell	160
Spanish	170
Granny Goose	168
Planters	170
Spanish, dry roasted	162
Peanut Crisps	150
Skippy	165
Tavern Nuts	171
Pecans	
A & P	200
Granny Goose	203
Planters	190
Pistachios	
Frito-Lay	174

Granny Goose	176
Planters	169
Sesame Mix	
Planters	163
Soybeans	
Malt-O-Meal	
dry roasted	132
oil roasted	141
Planters	133
Sunflower Seeds	
whole, 1 lb	1,371
whole, 1 cup	257
hulled, 1 cup	810

CHAPTER 13

Fast Foods and Snacks

CHIPS, PUFFS, CRISPS, ETC.

1 oz unless noted

Bows	163
Bugles	163
Buttons	147
Cheddar Bitz	
Frito-Lay	130
Cheese Doodles	
Old London	141
Cheese Pixies	
Wise	160

Cheese Twists	
Jax	136
Wonder	154
Cheetos	
Frito-Lay	158
Cheez Balls	
Planters	163
Cheez Curls	
Planters	163
Corn Chips	
Fritos	155
Barbecue	159
Granny Goose	159
Old London	151
Barbecue	149
Planters	170
Wise	165
Barbecue	150
Wonder	168
Corn Nuggets	
Frito-Lay	128
Clam Crisps	
Snow's	166
Fiesta Chips	
Granny Goose	146
Flings	
Nabisco	167
Swiss 'n Ham	148
Funyuns	138

Salted	121
Sesame	119
Whole wheat	122
Taco Chips	
Old London	127
Tortilla Chips	
Doritos	
Nachos	137
Tacos	142
Granny Goose	144
Planters	
Nachos	128
Tacos	132
Wheat Chips	
Bakon Snacks	147

PIZZA, FROZEN, 1 whole pizza unless noted

Beef and Cheese	
El Chico	
with enchilada	1,010
with taco	990
Bacon	
Tostino's	704

Cheese	
Buitoni	276
Celeste	473
large	1,280
Sicilian	1,395
with mushroom, small	459
with mushroom, large	1,205
Chef Boy-Ar-Dee	798
small	160
Jeno's	840
Deluxe	1,470
Junior	165
Mix	838
Kraft	822
Pee Wee	170
Lambrecht	909
La Pizzeria	1,230
Lean Cuisine	170
Roman	891
Stouffer's	330
Tostino's	882
Cheese and Refried Beans	
El Chico	902
Cheese and Chili	
El Chico	1,039
Combinations	
Celeste	600
large	1,480
Jeno's Deluxe	1,667

La Pizzeria	830
large	1,529
Stouffer's	789
Tostino's	1,683
Classic	1,675
Hamburger	
Jeno's	888
Tostino's	910
Crisp	955
Open Face	
Buitoni	250
Pepperoni	
Celeste	540
large	1,438
Chef Boy-Ar-Dee	175
Jeno's	901
La Pizzeria	1,322
Roman	889
Stouffer's	800
Tostino's	923
Crisp	960
Classic	1,792
Classic with mushrooms	1,497
Rolls	
Jeno's	
Cheeseburger	268
Pepperoni	262
Sausage	259
Shrimp	214

Sausage	
Celeste	561
large	1,500
Jeno's	899
Deluxe	1,495
Mix	1,058
Kraft	1,000
Pee Wee	190
Lambrecht	1,005
La Pizzeria	860
large	1,515
Roman	233
Tostino's	938
Crisp	981
Classic	1,799

POPCORN AND PRETZELS

Popcorn, 1 cup	
Jiffy Pop	31
Jolly Time	31
King Korn	
Cheese	40
Seasoned	42
Pops-Rite	38

Presto-Pop	37
3 Minute	38
TNT	52
Wise	43
Cheese-flavored	49
Wonder	45
Pretzels, 1 piece	
Bachman	
B's	8
Beer	55
Medium	20
Teeny	11
Thin	18
Old London	5
Nabisco Mister Salty	
Dutch	51
3-Ring	12
Veri-Thin	20
Pretzelettes	6
Sunshine	19

FAST FOODS

Arby's	
Beef and Cheese Sandwich	450
Club Sandwich	560

Ham and Cheese Sandwich	380
Junior Roast Beef Sandwich	220
Roast Beef Sandwich	350
Super Roast Beef Sandwich	620
Swiss King Sandwich	660
Turkey Deluxe Sandwich	510
Turkey Sandwich	410
Arthur Treacher's	
Chicken	271
Chicken Sandwich	265
Chips	243
Chowder	66
Cole Slaw	144
Fish	241
Fish Sandwich	282
Krunch Pup	358
Lemon Luvs	324
Shrimp	380
Brazier (Dairy Queen)	
Hamburger	260
Cheeseburger	320
Big Brazier	460
Big Brazier with Cheese	550
Big Brazier with Lettuce and Tomato	470
Super Brazier (The Half-Pounder)	780
Hot Dog	270
Hot Dog with Chili	330
Hot Dog with Cheese	330
Fish Sandwich	400
Fish Sandwich with Cheese	440

French Fries	200
French Fries, large	320
Onion Rings	300
Burger Chef	
Chocolate Shake	310
Big Chef	542
Cheeseburger	304
Double Cheeseburger	434
Double Hamburger	325
French Fries	187
Hamburger	258
Mariner Platter	680
Rancher Platter	640
Shake	326
Skipper's Treat	604
Super Chef	600
Burger King	
Whopper	650
Double Beef *Whopper*	850
Whopper with Cheese	760
Double Beef *Whopper* with Cheese	970
Whopper Junior	360
Whopper Junior with Cheese	420
Whopper Junior with Double Meat	490
Whopper Junior Double Meat with Cheese	550
Hamburger	310
Hamburger with Cheese	360
Double Meat Hamburger	440
Double Meat Hamburger with Cheese	540

Steak Sandwich	600
Whaler	660
Whaler with Cheese	770
Onion Rings, large	330
Onion Rings, regular	230
French Fries, large bag	360
French Fries, regular bag	240
Chocolate Milkshake	380
Vanilla Milkshake	360
Apple Pie	240
Carl's Jr.	
Famous Star Hamburger	480
Super Star Hamburger	660
Old Time Star Hamburger	440
Happy Star Hamburger	290
Steak Sandwich	630
California Roast Beef Sandwich	380
Fish Fillet Sandwich	550
Original Hot Dog	340
Chili Dog	360
Chili Cheese Dog	400
American Cheese	40
Salad with Condiments 11 oz	170
Dressing, 2 oz	
Blue Cheese	200
Thousand Island	190
Lo-Cal Italian	48
French Fries	220
Apple Turnover	330

Carrot Cake	380
Shake	310
Soft Drinks	200
***Church's Fried Chicken*, 1 piece, boned**	
Dark	305
White	327
Dunkin' Donuts	
Cake and Chocolate Cake Donuts	
rings, sticks, crullers, etc.	240
Yeast-raised Donuts	160
Glazed Yeast-Raised Donuts	168
Fancies	
coffee rolls, danish, etc.	215
Fancies with Filling and Topping	260
Munchkins, Yeast-raised	26
Munchkins, Cake and Chocolate Cake	66
Munchkins with Filling and Topping	79
Gino's	
Apple Pie	238
Cheeseburger	300
Cheese Hero	738
Cheese Sirloiner	532
Coke	117
Fish Platter	650
Fish Sandwich	450
French Fries	156
Giant	569
Hamburger	254
Hero	647
Hot Chocolate	90

Hardees	
Apple Turnover	282
Big Twin	447
Cheeseburger	335
Deluxe	675
Double Cheeseburger	495
Fish Sandwich	468
French Fries, large	381
French Fries, small	239
Hamburger	305
Hot Dog	346
Milkshake	391
Roast Beef Sandwich	390
Jack-in-the-Box	
Apple Turnover	411
Breakfast Jack	301
Cheeseburger	
Deluxe	310
Jumbo Jack	628
Double Cheese Omelet	423
French Fries	270
French Toast	537
Hamburger	
Bonus Jack	461
Deluxe	260
Jumbo Jack	551
Ham and Cheese Omelet	425
Jack Burrito	448
Jack Steak	428
Lemon Turnover	446

Moby Jack	455
Onion Rings	351
Pancakes	626
Ranchero Omelet	414
Scrambled Eggs	719
Shakes, Chocolate	365
Strawberry	380
Vanilla	342
Taco	189
Taco Super	285
Kentucky Fried Chicken	
Chicken Dinner	
(3 pieces chicken, potatoes, cole slaw, roll)	
Original Recipe Dinner	830
Extra Crispy Dinner	950
Individual Pieces	
Wing	151
Drumstick	136
Keel	253
Rib	242
Thigh	276
Long John Silver's	
Breaded Clams	465
Breaded Oysters	460
Chicken planks	458
Cole Slaw	138
Corn on the Cob	174
Fish with Batter, 2 pieces	318
Fries	375

Hush Puppies	153
Ocean Scallops	257
Peg Leg	514
Shrimp	268
Treasure Chest	467
McDonald's	
Apple Pie	300
Big Mac	541
Cheeseburger	306
Cherry Pie	298
Chocolate Shake	364
Egg McMuffin	352
English Muffin, Buttered	186
Fillet O' Fish	402
French Fries	211
Hamburger	257
Hot Cakes, with Butter or Syrup	472
McDonaldland Cookies	294
Quarter-pounder	418
Quarter-pounder with Cheese	518
Sausage	184
Scrambled eggs	162
Shake, Strawberry	345
Shake, Vanilla	323
***Pizza Hut*, 1 slice, Thin**	
Standard	
Cheese	180
Pepperoni	202
Pork and Mushroom	196

Super Supreme	266
Superstyle	
Cheese	213
Pepperoni	233
Pork and Mushroom	230
Supreme	216
***Ponderosa*, Entree**	
Chopped Beef	324
Double Deluxe	362
Extra-cut Prime Rib	409
Extra-cut Ribeye	358
Fillet of Sole	251
Fillet of Sole Sandwich	125
Junior Patty	98
Prime Rib	286
Ribeye	259
Ribeye/Shrimp	400
Shrimp	220
Steakhouse Deluxe	181
Strip Sirloin	277
Super Sirloin	383
T-Bone	374
Poppin' Fresh	
Chef's Salad	800
Custard Pie, 1 slice	380
Dairy Salad	650
Dinner Salad	250
Doughboy Salad	530
Pumpkin Pie, 1 slice	390

Shrimp Salad	640
Tuna Salad	640
Steak 'N Shake	
Steakburger	276
Steakburger with Cheese	352
Super Steakburger	375
Super Steakburger with Cheese	451
Triple Steakburger	474
Triple Steakburger with Cheese	625
Low Calorie Platter	293
Baked Ham Sandwich	451
Toasted Cheese Sandwich	250
Ham & Egg Sandwich	434
Egg Sandwich	275
French Fries	211
Chili and Oyster Crackers	337
Chili	402
Baked Beans	173
Lettuce and Tomato Salad with 1 oz Thousand Island Dressing	168
Chef Salad	313
Cottage Cheese	93
Apple Danish	391
Sundaes	
Strawberry	329
Hot Fudge Nut	530
Brownie Fudge	645
Apple Pie	407
Cherry Pie	334

Cheesecake	368
Brownie	259
Taco Bell	
Bean Burrito	343
Beef Burrito	466
Beefy Tostada	291
Bellbeefer	221
Bellbeefer with Cheese	278
Burrito Supreme	457
Combination Burrito	404
Enchirito	454
Pintos Cheese	168
Taco	186
Tostada	179
Wendy's	
Cheeseburger	
Single cheese	580
Double cheese	800
Triple cheese	1,040
Chili	230
French Fries	330
Frosty	390
Hamburger	
Single	470
Double	670
Triple	850
White Castle	
Cheeseburger	185
Fish	192

French Fries	225
Hamburger	160
Zantiago	
Burrito	345
Enchirito	391
Frijoles	231
Taco	146
Tostada	206

CHAPTER 14

Home Cooked, Restaurant and Frozen

HOME COOKED AND RESTAURANT DISHES,

1 average portion unless noted

Abalone with mushrooms	526
Abalone with oyster sauce	283
Abalone steaks	215
Aioli sauce, 1 Tbsp	125
Almond tarts, each	70
Alu Bhaji	130

Ambrosia	126
Ambrosia salad	542
Anchovy butter, 1 Tbsp	127
Angel Food Cake	120
Apples, baked	225
Apples, stuffed	265
Apple Brown Betty	547
Apples, candied	355
Apple Caramel	488
Apple cinnamon rings	180
Apple curried rings	155
Apple fried rings	165
Apple, pickled, 1 apple	50
Applesauce	225
Apple turnovers	400
Apricot, Brown Betty	498
Armenian style mussels, stuffed with rice, currants and piñon nuts	528
Arroz con Pollo	655
Artichoke, boiled	146
Artichoke hearts, marinated	75
Artichokes, Jerusalem boiled	163
Artichoke moutarde	374
Artichoke, Provencal-style, braised	127
Artichoke vinaigrette	446
Asparagus, buttered	90
Asparagus, Chinese-style	150
Asparagus Divan, 4 spears	375
Asparagus vinaigrette	170

Aspic	25
tomato	60
Athenian-style braised lamb shoulder	589
Austrian-style cabbage	210
Avgolemono sauce, 1 Tbsp	10
Avocado salad dressing, 1 Tbsp	63
Avocado salad, with Belgian endive	245
with tomato	288
farci, ½	400
de crabe, ½	410
de crevettes, ½	489
mousse	137
vinaigrette, ½	380
Baba Ghanouj, ½ cup	185
Bagel and lox with cream cheese	374
Bahamian style coffee	216
Bahamian style conch chowder	340
Baked Alaska	485
Baklava	350
Banana, baked	200
Banana, flambée	438
Banana tea bread	105
Bannock	119
Barbecued spareribs	500
Barley and mushroom casserole	300
Bavarian Cream	212
Bear, pot roasted	500
Béarnaise sauce, 1 Tbsp	48
Bechamel sauce, 1 Tbsp	36

Beef and Asparagus	929
and Bean Curd	682
and Bean Sprouts	646
and Broccoli	585
Congee	896
Consommé, 1 cup	33
Fondue Bourguignonne	479
and Green Pepper	444
Lo Mein	1,042
and Mushrooms	435
and Noodles in Brown Bean Sauce	685
and Oyster Sauce	689
with Pea Pods and Water Chestnuts	648
and Mushroom Pirog	720
Picadillo	400
Beef Brisket	530
Beef Heart, stuffed	475
Beef Kidneys, braised	275
Beef Roasts	
Pot-au-feu	555
Pot Roast	600
Pot Roast, French-style	715
Pot Roast, German-style	650
Sauerbraten	569
Yankee Pot Roast	746
Beef Short Ribs	485
Beef Steak	
Bracioulini	423
Chicken-fried	935
Chinese-style	345

Beets	
harvard in sour cream	170
in horseradish	120
pickled, 1 beet	10
Beignet d 'Aubergines, 4 oz	200
Beurre Manié, 1 Tbsp	98
Bhendi Bhaji	85
Bernaise Sauce, 1 Tbsp	46
Billi-Bi	222
Biscuit Tortoni	284
Biscuit, Baking Powder, 1 piece	83
Black Bean dip, 1 Tbsp	36
Black-eyed peas, Southern-style	550
Black forest cake	758
Blancmange	162
Blanquette de Veau	699
Blini, 1 piece	87
with butter	184
with caviar	204
Blintzes, cheese, 1 piece	177
Blood Sausage, 6 oz	708
Blueberry muffins	133
Blueberry waffles	259
Bocconcini	524
Bordelaise sauce, 1 Tbsp	23
Borscht	400
Boston Baked beans	534
Boston Brown Bread, 1 slice	86
Bougatsa, 1 piece	401
Bouillabaisse	600

Bourek, 1 piece	98
Brains with Almonds	653
braised	338
with sherry	570
Brandied Peaches, 1 peach	65
Bratwurst, grilled, 6 oz	500
Bratwurst, sauteed, 6 oz	563
Brandy Alexander pie	680
Brandy sauce, 1 Tbsp	44
hard, 1 Tbsp	115
Brandy snaps, 1 piece	98
Brazilian Black Beans	376
Bread sauce, 1 Tbsp	18
Brioche	201
Broccoli amandine	279
Broccoli with Parmesan	105
Brownie, 1 piece	160
Buche de Noel	684
Buffalo Steak, broiled	400
Bulgar, pilaf	290
plain	277
Buttermilk Biscuits, 1 piece	88
Buttermilk salad dressing, 1 Tbsp	9
Butterscotch Brownie, 1 piece	156
Butterscotch Sauce, 1 Tbsp	71
Burrito with Beans	321
with Chili	251
with Beef and Beans	335
Bytky	631

Food	Calories
Cabbage	
Austrian	227
Baked	106
Colcannon	144
Creole	133
Flemish Red, with Apples	268
Pennsylvania Dutch	155
Pickled, 1 cup	200
Polish	400
Rolls Stuffed with Lamb	372
Sweet and Sour	150
Cacciucco	414
Cacik	100
Caesar salad	299
Cake	
Applesauce	205
Cheesecake	424
Cheesecake, Italian style	520
Chocolate	230
Cinnamon and Coffee	135
Coconut cream	240
Devil's food	240
Lemon Chiffon	300
Light Fruit	266
Genoese	120
Marble	195
Petits fours, 1 piece	251
Pineapple Upside-down	255
Rainbow	210
Sachertorte	362

Spice	205
Sponge	100
Wedding	150
Trifle	585
Calamari, Baked	286
Calf's Liver	
sauteed	260
with Bacon	375
with Onions	310
alla Veneziana	310
Cannelloni with Beef	398
with Ricotta	356
with Spinach	397
Cannoli	190
Cantonese fried fish, 4 oz	449
Cantonese Lobster	400
Cantonese Shrimp and Vegetables	372
Capicola, 1 slice	108
Caponata, 1 Tbsp	18
Caramel popcorn ball, 1 piece	212
Carp, Sweet and Sour	332
in Brown Sauce	726
Caviar, 1 oz	89
Carrots with dill, 1 cup	55
Carrot tzimmes	707
Cassoulet	1,000
Catalan beef	776
Cauliflower au gratin	323
Cauliflower salad	180
Caviar au gratin, 2 oz	259

Celeri Rémoulade, 4 oz	303
Celeriac, creamed	213
Ceviche	308
Champ	157
Champignon farci gratinée, 1 piece	135
Chantilly Sauce, 1 Tbsp	75
Chard, pureed	107
Char shu ding	300
Charlotte Russe	458
Chasseur Sauce, 1 Tbsp	31
Cheese Boreks	138
Cheese Dumplings, 1 piece	95
Cheese Fondue	1,000
Cheese straws, 10 pieces	283
Cheese sauce, 1 Tbsp	38
Cheese souffle	327
Cherries Jubilee	200
Chestnuts	
creamed	400
pureed	327
roasted, 6 oz	245
Chicken	
and Almonds	750
and Asparagus	510
Barbecued with Skin and Bones	405
Bhuna	219
and Black Bean Sauce	748
Burmese, in Peanut and Coconut Sauce	845
Cacciatore	468
and Cashews	750

Chop Suey	355
Chow Mein	260
Circassian	950
Crispy Fried, Chinese-style	669
Coq au Vin Blanc	385
Coq au Vin Rouge	408
Creamed	426
Croquettes	440
Dahi	220
Dhan Sak	239
Diavolo	290
Divan	378
Drunken Chicken, Chinese	593
Foo Yong	434
Fricassee	469
Francese	320
Jade	666
Jaipur	795
Jambalaya	533
Kiev	520
a la King	390
Kung Pow	482
Lemon	796
Livers, sauteed	120
Lo Mein	728
Maglai	236
Magyar	457
Marengo	366
Moo Goo Gai Pan	248
Molé	562

Musallam	227
with Mushrooms	528
Pancake, Chinese-style	899
Parmigiana	510
Pizziola	290
Roumanian-style, with Apricots	468
Salad	423
with Snow peas	520
Stew	560
stuffed with rice and mushrooms	362
Sub Gum	638
Sweet and Sour	1,150
Tandoori	366
Teriyaki	878
Tetrazzini	878
Chinese-style, with vegetables	670
Velvet	742
Vino bianco	300
with walnuts	929
Yakitori	253
Zingara	500
and tomato salad	199
Chili	448
Chiles con Queso	327
Chiles Rellenos	442
Chiles de Frijoles	544
Chimichango	288
Chinese style	
Beef	343
Cabbage, quickfried	200

Cabbage, steamed	85
Cabbage, Sweet and Sour	200
Carp, Sweet and Sour	300
Mustard Sauce, 1 Tbsp	5
Egg roll	145
Fried eggs and Rice	324
Fried puffs, 1 piece	86
Fried rice	301
Pork with rice	277
Shrimp with ginger	274
Snow peas	115
Spareribs	565
Sweet and sour sauce, 1 Tbsp	15
Cucumber and soy sauce	62
Chocolate	
Chiffon Cake, 1 slice	318
Chip Cookie, 1 piece	75
Eclairs	282
Mousse	316
Profiteroles, 1 piece	153
Sauce, 1 Tbsp	86
Hot Soufflé	339
Chinese fried puffs, 1 piece	86
Chopped Chicken liver, ½ cup	262
Chorizos, 1 link	147
Chutney, 1 Tbsp	
Coconut	17
Green Tomato	25
Mango	63

Mint	10
Tomato	30
Clams	
Bisque	200
in Black Bean Sauce, Chinese-style, 1	39
Casino, 1 dozen	536
New England Pie	325
Origanata, 1 dozen	440
Red Sauce	301
White Sauce	142
Cockaleekie	95
Cocoa	175
Coconut Macaroon, 1 piece	57
Cod Kedgeree	333
Coleslaw and caraway salad	238
Court Bouillon	4
Couscous, Boiled	305
Beef	567
Chicken	653
Lamb	600
Coquilles Saint-Jacques	475
Cornbread, 1 slice	100
Corn Fritters	249
relish, 1 Tbsp	16
sticks, per stick	100
Corned beef and cabbage	600
Corned beef hash	400
Coulibiac	288
Crab	
Cakes, Maryland-style	257

Cocktail, ½ cup	92
Deviled	398
Legs, Alaska King	297
Louis	767
Meunière, 2	278
Mornay	513
Newburg Imperial	426
Cranberry Nut Bread, 1 slice	136
Cranberry Relish, 1 Tbsp	44
Cranberry sauce, 1 Tbsp	28
Cream Cheese Dip, with Bacon and Horseradish, 1 Tbsp	74
Cream Puff, 1 piece	251
Creme brulee	655
Creme Caramel	280
Crepes, au champignon, 1 piece	178
Crepes, au jambon gratinée, 1 piece	156
Crepes Suzette, 1 piece	208
Crispy Bass, Chinese-style	484
Croissant, 1 piece	90
Croque Madame	710
Croque Monsieur	710
Croquettes de crevette	263
Croquettes de volaille	493
Cucumber and yogurt sauce, 1 Tbsp	5
Crumpet, 1 piece	80
Cumberland sauce, 1 Tbsp	40
Curried	
Beef	415
Beef Triangles, 1 piece	154

Lamb	656
Lamb and dhal	870
Cold lobster	493
Shrimp	504
Custard, baked	**162**
Custard, floating island	**253**
Custard, rennet	**107**
Custard sauce	**27**
Danish pastry	**144**
Datenut bread, 1 slice	**88**
Dhal	**229**
Deviled Ham, 1 Tbsp	**38**
Diable sauce, 1 Tbsp	**20**
Dijonnaise sauce, 1 Tbsp	**93**
Dips, 1 Tbsp	
Black bean	37
Chili	18
Clam in Cream Cheese	75
Cream cheese, bacon and horseradish	71
Curry	40
Deviled clam	80
Taramasalata	102
Divinity, 1 piece	**38**
Dolma	**225**
Doughnut	
chocolate, 1 piece	175
jelly	147
old fashioned	135
Duck	
with Cherry sauce	400

Crispy, Chinese style, 4 oz	820
Eight precious, 4 oz	905
with Orange sauce	490
Peking, 4 oz	835
Pressed, 4 oz	399
Wild roast	256
Szechuan, 4 oz	1,000
Tangerine peel, Chinese-style	782
Dumplings, Chinese-style, 1 piece	95
Dumplings, Peking fried, 1 piece	76
Duxelles sauce, 1 Tbsp	19
East Indian Lentils and Rice	264
Eclairs, 1 piece	285
Eel, jellied	605
Eel and egg pie	623
Eggs	
in Aspic, 1	130
Benedict, 1	286
Custard, steamed Chinese-style	226
Deviled, 1	148
Florentine, 1	165
Foo Yong, 1 foo	322
Fried rice, 1 cup	335
Huevos rancheros, 1	177
Salad	403
Scotch, 1	498
Eggnog, nonalcoholic	243
Eggplant	
Basque-style with peppers and tomatoes	155
Dip, 1 Tbsp	45

Fried	281
Greek-style	195
Greek-style, stuffed	180
Ismir	246
Parmigiana	598
Pisto	135
Ratatouille	510
Stuffed with mushrooms and chickpeas	228
Stuffed with pilaf and raisins	188
Turkish	327
Egg Rolls, Chinese, 1 piece	145
Empanada, with beef	244
Empanada, with chicken	220
Enchilada	
Beef	299
Cheese	270
Chicken	330
Chorizo	267
Escalopes de veau cordon bleu	680
Escargot de bourgogne, 6 pieces	418
Escarole, sautéed	74
Esterhazy steak	994
Falafel	263
Fennel, braised	116
Fettuccine Alfredo	1,550
Fettuccine con Baccala	653
Figs, fresh stewed	195
Finnan Haddie	257
Fish balls, Chinese-style, 8 oz	319

Fish, Jade Chinese-style, 6 oz	547
Lemon Chinese-style, 8 oz	754
Fish mousse	286
Fish piquant en papillote	199
Fish soufflé	300
Flan	263
Flemish red cabbage and apples	248
Floating island	257
Florentines, 1 piece	118
Flounder fillet in black bean sauce	600
Fondue de Gruyère	478
Fragrant noodles with shrimp, Chinese-style	810
Franks in blankets, 1 piece	46
French-fried onion rings	165
French-fried potatoes	227
Frijoles fritos	325
Frijoles Mexicanos	194
Frikadeller	384
Fruit cake, light, 1 slice	264
Fudge, chocolate, 1 piece	78
Fudge Sauce, hot, 1 Tbsp	100
Garlic bread, 1 slice	88
Garlic sauce, 1 Tbsp	11
Gefilte fish	183
Giblet gravy, 1 Tbsp	16
Gingersnaps, 1 piece	97
Gingerbread, 1 slice	206
Gingerbread boys, 1 boy	132
Gnocchi, Cheese	410

Farina parmigiana	385
Potato	314
Goose, Braised with chestnuts and onions	525
German style stuffed with potatoes	488
Roasted with apples and sauerkraut stuffing	842
Goulash	394
Grand Marnier soufflé	262
Grand Marnier with strawberries	110
Granite, 1 cup	263
Grasshopper pie	680
Gravy, 1 Tbsp	
au jus	4
giblet	15
mushroom	22
Greek Salad	235
Greek Gyro	246
Green Olives, 2 large	20
Green Beans with garlic, Chinese-style	205
Green Goddess dressing, 1 Tbsp	89
Grenouilles a l'Anglaise	385
Meuniere	485
Provencale	423
Green pepper, Stuffed	190
with beef and kidney beans	356
Mexican-style	444
Green sauce, 1 Tbsp	82
Grits	150
Guacamole, 1 Tbsp	28
Gumbo, corn	172

Gumbo, shrimp	308
Haddock, Baked	300
Creamy smoked and potato casserole	425
Ham	
in aspic	600
fried with red eye gravy	400
loaf	427
Tetrazzini	590
Hamburger	
bacon	400
broiled	280
cheese	370
chili	285
Pizza	285
mushroom	270
Hash	310
Hawaiian spareribs	409
Herb Butter, 1 Tbsp	125
Herring	
and beets a la Russe	591
in dill sauce	188
in mustard sauce	150
in oatmeal	370
Pickled	217
Rollmops	239
Scandanavian salad	379
in sour cream	127
Hoagie, 1 roll	400
Hog Jowl and Black-Eyed Peas	351
Hollandaise sauce, 1 Tbsp	48

Horseradish cream sauce, 1 Tbsp	**77**
Horseradish, fresh, 1 Tbsp	**5**
Hot Chocolate	**275**
Hot Cross Bun, 1 piece	**105**
Huevos Rancheros, 1 egg	**186**
Humus with tahini, ½ cup	**364**
Hushpuppies, 1 piece	**67**
Indian Corn Fritters, 1 piece	**50**
Indian Pudding	**371**
Indian Rice Pilaf	**395**
Irish Soda Bread, 1 slice	**114**
Irish Stew	**710**
Japanese Salad	
autumn	**150**
cucumber	**48**
cucumber and fish	**135**
cucumber and seaweed	**64**
lotus root	**87**
Jelly, homemade, 1 Tbsp	**45**
Jelly Roll	**187**
Jhinga Bhajia, 1 piece	**37**
Jhinga Kari, 10-12 shrimp	**609**
Jhonnycake, 1 piece	**98**
Kasha, buckwheat	**355**
appel-almond	**400**
Katsudon	**829**
Kebabs, Indian lamb	**231**
Kedgeree	**318**
Keema curry	**246**
Keftedakia Marinata	**410**

Keftedes	**248**
Keftedes Avgolemono	**200**
Khiri Pachadi	**122**
Kibbeh	**964**
Kidneys, braised	**289**
Kielbasa, fried, 3 oz	**350**
Kissel	**240**
Knockwurst, sauteed, 6 oz	**538**
Korma curry	**344**
Koulebiaka	**1,300**
Kourabiedes, 1 piece	**75**
Kreplach, 1 piece	**34**
Kugelhupf, 1 slice	**187**
Ladyfingers, 1 piece	**52**
Lamb	
braised	**490**
breast	**425**
cassoulet	**1,050**
crown roast	**270**
dolma	**232**
kidneys in sour cream	**485**
riblets, barbecued	**840**
shanks	**372**
shish kebab	**686**
stew	**403**
Lancashire Hot Pot	**552**
Lasagne, with cheese	**605**
with meat	**408**
with meat balls	**1,095**
Lebkuchen, 1 piece	**84**

Leek pie	562
Lemon curd, 1 Tbsp	50
Lemonade	118
Lemon Ice	140
Lemon sauce, 1 Tbsp	28
Lemon Sherbet, 1 cup	290
Lentils, boiled	364
Linguini alla Romana	763
Linzertorte, Viennese, 1 slice	304
Liver, Broiled	280
and onions	306
alla Veneziana	314
Chicken, sautéed	247
Chicken pâté	294
Lo mein pork	333
Lobster	
a l'Americaine	503
Cantonese	393
Fra diavolo	586
Mousse	300
Newburg	483
Thermidor	483
London Broil	389
Lotus Root Cake	70
Louisiana Rice and Kidney Beans	483
Lyonnaise sauce, 1 Tbsp	31
Macaroni, Beef and Tomato Casserole	656
and cheese	482
salad	471
Macaroon, 1 piece	44

Mácedoine of vegetables	**155**
Madeira wine sauce, 1 Tbsp	**29**
Madeleines, 1 piece	**40**
Mandel Torte	**523**
Mannicotti with cheese	**275**
Mannicotti with meat	**292**
Maquereau au vin blanc, 4 oz	**192**
Marinara sauce, 1 cup	**200**
Marshmellow cream sauce, 1 Tbsp	**49**
Marzipan, 1 piece	**87**
Matzo balls, 1 piece	**21**
Mayonnaise, 1 Tbsp	**130**
Meatballs	
Danish	**396**
hot and spicy	**158**
Konigsberger klops	**573**
Savory	**399**
Swedish	**693**
Lamb stuffed with bulgar	**335**
Turkish lamb baked in tomato sauce	**556**
Meat Loaf, plain	**222**
Meat Loaf, spicy	**621**
Melba sauce, 1 Tbsp	**34**
Meringue, 1 piece	**47**
Meringue Chantilly, 1 piece	**196**
Milkshake	**569**
Mincemeat Pie, brandied	**588**
Mint sauce, 1 Tbsp	**25**
Molasses Cookies, 1 piece	**58**
Molé sauce, 1 Tbsp	**24**

Moo goo gai pan	244
Mornay sauce, 1 Tbsp	33
Moules	
farcis provencale, 8–10 pieces	324
gratinées Normande, 8–10 pieces	285
Marseille, 8–10 pieces	450
salade de, 8–10 pieces	461
vinaigrette, 8–10 pieces	230
Moussaka	818
Mousse, Avocado	196
Chocolate	306
Fish	282
Mozzarella cheese, breaded and fried	231
Muffin, 1 piece	108
Bran	140
Corn	148
Raisin bran	162
Mushroom gravy, 1 Tbsp	26
Mushrooms	
creamed	200
in madeira	236
marinated	51
sauteed	187
Mushrooms with bamboo shoots	295
Mu shu pork, 2 pancakes	874
Mustard sauce, 1 Tbsp	41
Nachos, 1 piece	40
Nantua sauce, 1 Tbsp	24
Napoleons, 1 piece	402

Napolitos	100
New England boiled dinner	735
Nockerln	163
Noodles in brown bean sauce and pork	891
Noodles in oyster sauce	463
Normandy rock cornish game hen, 1 bird	700
Oatmeal Bread, 1 slice	120
Octopus Mediterranean	350
Okra, fried	175
Omelet	
with caviar, 1 egg	180
Greek, 1 egg	130
Lorraine, 1 egg	167
Lyonnaise, 1 egg	136
with mushroom and tomato, 1 egg	135
Onion frittata, 1 egg	200
Piperade, 1 egg	215
Soufflé, 1 egg	111
Spanish, 1 egg	127
Onion Rings, french-fried	184
Onions, baked, 1 piece	155
Onions, creamed	209
sautéed	150
stuffed	186
Oshi tashi	34
Osso buco	905
Oysters casino, 1 dozen	540
Oysters en Brochette	215
Oysters Rockefeller, 1 dozen	1,000

Oyster Sauce, 1 Tbsp	35
Paella	
with lobster	620
with sausage	630
Valenciana	548
Pakora (Indian fritters)	
Baigon	41
Gobhi	38
Mixed vegetable	54
Pancakes, 1 piece	
apple	95
blueberry	87
buckwheat	82
buttermilk	73
pecan	135
plain	85
wholewheat	89
Panettone, 1 slice	322
Paper-wrapped Chicken, Chinese-style, 1 piece	98
Parsley sauce, 1 Tbsp	22
Parsnips, roasted	211
Pashka	300
Pastitsio	820
Pâté	
de Campagne	584
de Canard	1,076
de Foie Gras	648
de Poisson au Asperges	478
Peach	
cardinal	230

cobbler	500
Melba	354
Peanut brittle, 1 piece	77
Peanut butter cookies, 1 piece	70
Pea pods with water chestnuts	307
Pea pods with mushrooms	261
Pear Helene	602
Peking custard	464
Penuche, 1 piece	41
Pepper, Greek stuffed green	120
Pepper, Greek stuffed with rice	160
Peppermint sauce, 1 Tbsp	46
Pepperoni, 1 slice	26
Pfeffernusse, 1 piece	82
Picadillo	400
Piccalilli, 1 Tbsp	12
Pie	
Apple, country	410
Apple, deep dish	445
Banana Cream	626
Blueberry	475
Boston Cream	265
Chocolate cream	610
Coconut cream	462
Coconut custard	400
Key Lime	693
Lemon Meringue	545
Nesselrode	516
Peach	400
Pecan	585

Pumpkin	400
Shoofly	528
Pigeon Pie	587
Pig's feet, 1 foot	251
Pigs in blanket	200
Pilaf	
Bulgur	306
Lamb	572
Rice	312
Piquante sauce, 1 Tbsp	19
Pirog, Beef and Mushroom	727
Piroshki	155
Pissaladiere	474
Pita bread	247
Pizza, 1 slice	
Plain	450
Green peppers	452
Mushrooms	462
Pepperoni	587
Plantains	136
Plum pudding, Steamed	451
Plum sauce, 1 Tbsp	30
Polenta	88
Pollo en Salsa verde	244
Pollo molé verde	367
Popcorn balls, 1 ball	249
Poppy seed bread sticks, 1 piece	18
Pork	
Balls, steamed, Chinese-style	488
Barbecued	357

Barbecued with vegetables, Chinese-style	640
Breaded, Italian-style	423
Choucroute garnie	1,000
with rice, Spanish-style	481
Crown roast	584
Loin, stuffed with apples and prunes	685
Lo mein	849
Red, cooked with chestnuts, Chinese-style	432
Sliced, Chinese-style	306
Sliced with green pepper, Chinese-style	411
Soong	666
Spareribs, barbecued	415
Spareribs, Chinese	555
Stuffed with oysters	400
Subgum chow mein	322
Suckling pig	1,100
Sweet and sour, Chinese-style	643
Sweet and sour stew	629
Szechuan-style with bean curd	576
Tenderloin, roast	345
Twice cooked in brown sauce	625
Twice cooked in Hoisin sauce	548
Teriyaki	453
Portugese Filhos, 1 piece	45
Potato Bread, 1 slice	70
Potatoes	
Anna	186
Au Gratin	310
Dauphine	268
Duchess	209

French-fried	232
Hash Brown	230
Lyonnaise	289
Pancakes	144
Potage Saint-Germain	102
Rosti	162
Salad	475
Salad, German-style	270
Scalloped	215
Pot-au-feu	547
Poulet	
a l'Estragon	435
Bonne Femme	410
Cordon Bleu	502
Roti Chasseur	428
Roti Normande	463
Pound Cake, 1 slice	363
Pralines, 1 piece	173
Profiteroles, 1 piece	97
Prosciutto and melon	120
Pudding	
Bread and butter	258
Chocolate	312
Indian	374
Plum, steamed	442
Rice	255
Tapioca	220
Pumpernickel Bread, 1 slice	84
Quenelles, Chicken	493
Fish	148

Lyonnaise	481
Quiche	
Florentine	479
Lorraine	631
Nicoise	471
Onion	479
Rabbit	
Hasenpfeffer	369
with juniper berries	666
stew	458
Radish salad	100
Raisin Bread, 1 slice	115
Raita	48
Raspberry Mousse	565
Raspberry Sherbet	367
Ratatouille	510
Ravioli, cheese	642
Ravioli, meat	583
Remoulade dressing, 1 Tbsp	112
Rhubarb pie	494
Rice, plain, boiled, 1 cup	210
mushroom rice	400
Pilaf, plain	297
Risi e Bisi	365
Risotto	323
Risotto al burro	356
Risotto alla Milanese	300
Risotto al sugo	402
Risotto piselli	422
Sticks, 1 cup	436

Subgum, fried, 1 cup	436
Roghan Josh	278
Roquefort dressing, 1 Tbsp	71
Rum Custard	208
Rum sauce, 1 Tbsp	36
Russian dressing, 1 Tbsp	80
Rutabaga, boiled	153
Rye Bread, 1 slice	64
Sachertorte	363
Salad	
Caesar	302
Chef's	413
de Saucisson	410
Green Bean	185
Nicoise	305
Spinach with bacon dressing	147
Tabbouleh	262
Three Bean	310
Waldorf	888
Salami, Italian, 1 slice	87
Salisbury Steak	583
Salmon	
Fume au natural	154
Loaf	230
mousse	312
poached	426
soufflé	335
Salsa, 1 cup	253
Salsa Verde, 1 cup	120
Salsify, creamed	237

Saltimbocca	520
Sandwiches	
Bacon, lettuce, and tomato	268
Bagel with cream cheese	255
Bagel with lox and cream cheese	355
Bologna	355
Cheese, grilled	400
Cheese, grilled with bacon	543
Cheese, grilled with tomato	415
Chopped liver	382
Corned beef	446
Fried egg	225
Lobster salad	255
Meatball with tomato sauce	400
Meatloaf	300
Monte Cristo	920
Pastrami	560
Roast beef, overstuffed	490
Reuben	582
Salami	394
Shrimp salad	250
Steak	353
Tongue, overstuffed	475
Tuna fish salad	324
Turkey club	505
Sangria	93
Sardine Fraiches Marines, 4 oz	328
Sashimi, assorted, 4 oz	100
tako, 4 oz	87
Sate	500

Sauce Supreme, 1 Tbsp	34
Saucisson rémoulade	631
Sauerbraten	570
Sauerkraut, with juniper berries, braised	257
with caraway seeds	72
Sausage and Peppers, 2 pieces	882
Scallops, broiled	210
en Brochette	254
Scampi	178
Scrapple	288
Scungilli marinara	269
Sfogliatelli	244
Shabu-shabu	448
Shepherd's Pie	500
Shish kebab	679
Shortbread, Scottish	152
Shortcake, strawberry	591
Shrimp	
Ajillo, 8 large	466
in almond sauce, 8 large	333
Balls, Chinese-style	286
Batter-fried, Chinese-style, 1 piece	84
with bean curd, 12 medium	980
with black bean sauce, Chinese-style	464
Braised, Chinese-style 12 medium	905
Butterfly, Japanese-style	250
with cashews	536
creole	344
Egg foo yong	356
Fried in shell, Chinese-style, 12 medium	674

Glass	299
in green sauce, Spanish-style 8–10	290
Gumbo	327
Jumbalaya	500
in lobster sauce, Chinese-style, 12 medium	1,250
lo mein	501
with Mexican Chilis, 8–10	401
Newburg	600
One shrimp two flavors, 14 medium	900
Scampi	180
Stir-fried, 12 medium	738
Shu Mai, 1 piece	45
Sweet and sour, 12 medium	1,900
Szechuan pepper	324
Toast, 1 piece	162
Sloppy Joe	318
Snails a la bourguignonne, 1 dozen	320
Snails a la provencale, 1 dozen	300
Sole À L'Américaine	305
Amandine	509
Bonne femme	550
with Crab Sauce	300
Goujons de	460
Meuniere	490
Veronique	600
Sopapilla	128
Sopapilla with honey and cream	209
Soubise sauce, 1 Tbsp	20
Soufflé	
au fromage	197

a l'Orange	330
au Marrons	358
de Homard	187
de jambon	234
de Saumon	224
Florentine	140
Soups	
Almond, cream of	437
Artichoke	110
Asparagus	130
Asparagus, cream of	230
Avgolemono	150
Black bean	300
Cappelletti	206
Caraway	121
Cheddar Cheese	372
Chinese-style	
Abalone	128
Bean curd	42
Beef congee	255
Bird's nest	275
Chicken congee	301
Egg drop	89
Fish congee	137
Hot and sour	275
Rice	402
Shark's fin	288
Winter melon	187
Won ton	100
Clam chowder, Manhattan	163

Clam chowder, New England	283
Chicken noodle	78
Chicken and rice	78
Chicken with bean curd, Japanese-style	74
Consommé	42
Escarole	138
Garlic	197
Gazpacho	192
Hungarian cherry	375
Hungarian cream of barley	204
Minestrone	243
Miso with bean curd	79
Miso with fish balls	142
Mulligatawny	304
Mushroom, cream of	272
Oxtail	329
Pastina	134
Peanut, cream of	520
Potato	209
Pumpkin	150
Sauerkraut	128
Senegalese	314
Stracciatelli	125
Stschy	167
Tortellini	210
Turtle, home style	278
Vegetable, cream of	340
Sour cream and chive, 1 Tbsp	29
Sour Dough Bread, 1 slice	65
Souvlaki	291

Spaghetti, 1 cup	
Alfredo	405
Bolognese	357
with butter, cream and parmesan	401
Carbonara	860
Clam sauce, red	300
Clam sauce, white	344
Fagioli	348
with meatballs in sauce	853
Paglia e fieno	506
al pesto	980
Pomodoro	268
with sausage	471
Spatzle	165
Spiedini with anchovy	386
Spinach au gratin	275
Spinach, creamed	144
Spoon bread	632
Spumoni, 1 cup	510
Squid, Mediterranean	390
Stuffed with Rice, Greek-style	354
Squirrel Stew	500
Steamed Chinese sausage	778
Steamed Scallops with cabbage, Chinese-style, 8 pieces	300
Steamed Whole Fish, Chinese-style, 1 lb	902
Stifado	228
Stollen, 1 slice	145
Strawberries Romanoff	322
Strawberry Shortcake	500

Strudel	
Almond	398
Apple	360
Cheese	410
Cherry	405
Poppy seed	400
Stuffing, 1 cup	
Chestnut and mushroom	472
Corn bread	700
Herbed	210
Rice	263
Sage and onion	220
Submarine, 1 roll	381
Sukiyaki	348
Sushi	
Chirashi	460
Norimaki	468
Tekka maki	400
Sweet and Sour Chinese meatballs	936
Sweet and Sour fish, 1 lb	902
Sweet and Sour sauce, 1 Tbsp	20
Tabbouleh	304
Tacos	
Bean	275
Cheese	205
Chicken	245
Chili	348
Chorizo	367
Taffy, 1 piece	50
Tahini sauce, ¼ cup	167

Tamale pie	268
Tandoori fish	300
Shrimp, 10–12	288
Taramasalata, 1 Tbsp	100
Tartar sauce, 1 Tbsp	92
Tarte au champignon	382
au Oignons	570
Tea Eggs, 1 egg	85
Tempura	590
Tempura sauce, 1 Tbsp	5
Teriyaki	
Beef	213
Chicken	380
Pork	462
Teriyaki sauce, 1 Tbsp	15
Toad in the Hole	700
Toast, French, 1 slice	143
Toll House Cookies, 1 piece	60
Tomato Aspic	73
Tomatos, broiled	126
Tomato sauce, 1 Tbsp	10
Bolognese, 1 cup	330
Italian-style, 1 cup	215
with red clam, 1 cup	300
Tomatos, stewed	43
Tortellini with butter and parmesan	582
with ricotta and cream	600
Tortillas, 1 piece, plain	75
Chili	196
Chorizo	500

Tostada	
Beef	467
Chicken	443
Chicken with guacamole	319
Refried beans	411
Tripe and Onions	375
Truit fume au natural	136
Turkey congee, 1 cup	274
Turkey, creamed	440
Turkey Tetrazzini	895
Turnips, glazed	247
au Gratin	236
roast	142
Veal	
blanquette de vean	638
a la bourguignonne	440
Cutlet a la creme	580
Cutlet Milanese	293
Cutlet parmigiana	448
Cutlet valdostana	348
Marengo	543
Osso buco	926
Paprika	577
Parmigiana	478
and peppers	562
Piccate	333
Saltimbocca	520
Scaloppine	472
Schnitzel	437
Stuffed with prosciutto	485

Sweetbreads	
braised	300
creamed	535
with mushrooms	575
sauteed	200
with sherry	585
Terrine of Veal and Ham	250
Vitello Tonnata	850
a la zingara	602
Venison Burgers	360
Ragout of	437
Roast saddle of	205
Vichyssoise	410
Vinaigrette, 1 Tbsp	100
Weiner Schnitzel	415
a la Holstein	457
White sauce, 1 cup	400
Wild Boar, pot roast	500
Wild Duck, roasted	265
Won ton, fried sweet, 1 piece	59
Yakinasu, 4 oz	38
Yakitori	263
Yakitori donburi	781
Yam, candied	315
Yankee pot roast	775
Yogurt kholodnyk	40
Yogurt sauce, 1 Tbsp	9
Yorkshire Pudding	78
Yorkshire Scones, 1 piece	150
Yudofu	83

Zabaglione	177
Zeppole, 1 piece	42
Zucchini, Fried, 1 strip	37
Italian style	100
Sautéed, ½ cup	71
Zuppa di pesce	458
Zuppa Inglese	378

FROZEN DINNERS,

1 complete dinner (see also pp 141-144 and pp 150-153)

Beans and Franks	
Banquet	591
Morton	530
Swanson	550
Beef	
Banquet	312
Chopped	443
La Choy	342
Lean Cuisine Oriental	280
Morton	270
Chopped	340

Country Table	540
Steak House	920
Swanson	370
3-Course	490
Chopped	460
Hungry Man	540
Hungry Man 18 oz	730
Weight Watchers 10 oz	387
Weight Watchers 16 oz	586
Beef and Beans	
Swanson	500
Beef Stroganoff	
Stouffer's	390
Chicken	
La Choy	354
Morton	240
Swanson boneless	730
Weight Watchers	330
Chicken and Biscuits	
Green Giant	200
Chicken Croquettes	
Morton	410
Chicken Cacciatore	
Stouffer's	313
Weight Watchers	356
Chicken and Dumplings	
Banquet	282
Morton	280
Chicken, fried	
Banquet	530

Man Pleaser	1,026
Morton	470
Country Table	710
Swanson	570
3-Course	630
Hungry Man	620
Hungry Man, 15¼ oz	910
Hungry Man, Barbecue	760
Crispy Fried	650
Chicken, glazed	
Lean Cuisine	270
Chicken with noodles	
Morton	260
Chicken, oriental	
Weight Watchers	320
Chicken Parmigiana and Spinach	
Weight Watchers	200
Chicken and vegetables	
Lean Cuisine	260
Chop Suey	
Banquet	282
Chow Mein	
Banquet	282
Green Giant	130
Lean Cuisine	240
Enchilada	
Banquet	
Beef	479
Cheese	459
El Chico	680

Swanson	570
Van de Kamp	
Beef	420
Cheese	430
Fish	
Banquet	382
Haddock	419
Perch	434
Lean Cuisine	200
Morton	270
Weight Watchers	
Flounder	240
Haddock	250
Perch	320
Sole	240
Turbot	490
Fish and Chips	
Swanson	450
Hungry Man	760
Ham	
Banquet	369
Morton	440
Swanson	380
Hash	
Banquet	372
Italian	
Banquet	446
Swanson	420
Lasagna	
Lean Cuisine Zucchini Lasagne	260

Lean Line	270
Swanson	740
Macaroni and beef	
Banquet	394
Morton	260
Swanson	400
Macaroni and cheese	
Banquet	326
Morton	320
Swanson	390
Manicotti	
Lean Line	270
Meat Loaf	
Banquet	412
Morton	340
Country Table	480
Swanson	530
Meatball	
Swanson	400
Mexican	
Banquet	571
Combination	571
El Chico	820
Swanson	600
Pepper	
La Choy	349
Polynesian	
Swanson	490
Pork	
Swanson	470

Queso	
El Chico	810
Salisbury Steak	
Banquet	390
Morton	290
Country Table	430
Swanson	790
3-Course	490
Hungry Man	870
Saltillo	
El Chico	790
Sausage with veal, 1 link	
Lean Line	90
Stuffed Shells	
Lean Line	260
Shrimp	
La Choy	325
Spaghetti with beef	
Lean Cuisine	280
Spaghetti and meatball	
Banquet	450
Morton	360
Swanson	410
Hungry Man	660
Swiss Steak	
Swanson	350
Tacos, beef	
El Chico	410
Turkey	
Banquet	293

Man Pleaser	620
Morton	350
Country Table	600
Swanson	360
3-Course	520
Hungry Man	740
Weight Watchers	400
Veal Parmigiana	
Banquet	421
Morton	330
Swanson	520
Hungry Man	910
Weight Watchers	230
Western	
Banquet	417
Morton	410
Swanson	460
Hungry Man	890
Ziti, baked	
Lean Line	270

CHAPTER 15

Fingertip Low Calorie Guide

OVER 350 CALORIES

Frozen entrees (at less than 30 calories per ounce)

Banquet Buffet Supper Beef and Noodles, 32 oz	754
Banquet Buffet Supper Beef Stew, 32 oz	700
Banquet Buffet Supper Chicken and Noodles, 32 oz	764
Banquet Buffet Supper Beef sliced with gravy, 32 oz	782
Banquet Buffet Supper Turkey, 32 oz	564
La Choy Chicken	354

Morton Country Table Salisbury Steak, 15 oz	430
Swanson Hungry-Man Turkey, 13¼ oz	380
Weight Watchers Turkey Tetrazzini, 13 oz	380

200-350 CALORIES

Frozen entrees (at less than 30 calories per ounce)

Beef	
Banquet, 11 oz	312
Lean Cuisine, 9⅛ oz	280
Morton, 10 oz	270
Chicken	
Morton, 10 oz	240
Stouffer's	
Chicken a la King, 9½ oz	330
Creamed Chicken, 6½ oz	300
Chicken Divan, 8½ oz	335
Weight Watchers, 15 oz	330
Chicken and Biscuits	
Green Giant, 7 oz	200
Chicken Creole	
Weight Watchers, 13 oz	250
Chicken and Dumplings	
Banquet, 12 oz	282
Morton, 11 oz	280

Chicken with Noodles	
Green Giant, 9 oz	250
Morton, 10½ oz	260
Chicken Oriental	
Weight Watchers, 16 oz	320
Chicken Parmigiana and Spinach	
Weight Watchers, 9 oz	200
Chicken and Vegetables	
Lean Cuisine, 12¾ oz	260
Chicken White Meat with Peas	
Weight Watchers, 9 oz	270
Chop Suey	
Banquet, 12 oz	282
Chow Mein	
Banquet, 12 oz	282
Lean Cuisine, 11¼ oz	240
Eggplant Parmigiana	
Weight Watchers, 13 oz	280
Fish	
Lean Cuisine, 9 oz	200
Morton, 9 oz	270
Weight Watchers	
Flounder, 16 oz	240
Haddock, 16 oz	250
Perch, 16 oz	320
Sole, 16 oz	240
Sole with peas, mushrooms and lobster sauce, 9½ oz	200
Green Peppers with Beef	
Green Giant, 7 oz	200

Lasagne
Lean Line, 10 oz 270
Lasagne, Zucchini
Lean Cuisine, 11 oz 260
Macaroni with Beef
Green Giant, 9 oz 240
Morton, 10 oz 260
Macaroni and Cheese
Banquet, 12 oz 326
Morton, 11 oz 320
Manicotti
Lean Line, 11 oz 270
Salisbury Steak
Banquet, 11 oz 390
Morton, 11 oz 290
Shells, Stuffed
Lean Line, 11 oz 260
Spaghetti with Beef
Lean Cuisine, 11½ oz 280
Turkey
Banquet,11 oz 293
Swanson Turkey Slices, 8¾ oz 260
Ziti, Baked
Lean Line, 10 oz 270
Ziti with Veal and sauce
Weight Watchers, 13 oz 350
Veal Parmigiana with Zucchini
Weight Watchers, 9½ oz 230

Canned Entrees (at less than 30 calories per ounce)

Pasta, one can	
Ravioli	
Franco-American Beef, 7½ oz	220
Rotini	
Franco-American, 7½ oz	200
Macaroni	
Franco-American, 7½ oz	220
Macaroni and Meatballs	
Franco-American, 7½ oz	220
Meat, one can	
Beef Goulash	
Hormel, 7½ oz	240
Ham, whole	
Hormel, 6 oz	312
Tuna, in water, drained	
Chicken of the Sea solid white, 7 oz can	216

Fish, Fresh

Crab, steamed, meat only, 8 oz	211
Haddock, fillets, 8 oz	180
Halibut, fillets, 8 oz	226
Oysters, Pacific and Western, meat only, 8 oz	207

15 Meat

Beef

Chuck
- boneless, lean only, braised, 4 oz 219
- boneless, lean only, stewed, 4 oz 243

Flank steak, boneless, all lean, braised, 4 oz 222
ground, lean with 10% fat, 4 oz 203
porterhouse steak with 9% bone, lean only, broiled, 4 oz without bone 254
round steak, boneless, lean only, braised or broiled, 4 oz 296
sirloin steak, 7% bone, lean only, broiled, 4 oz without bone 235
T-bone, 11% bone, lean only, broiled, 4 oz without bone 253

Ham

fresh, lean only
- baked, without bone and skin, 4 oz 246

light cured, lean only
- baked, without bone and skin, 4 oz 328

Lamb

Leg, lean only, roasted, boneless, 4 oz 211
loin chops, with bone, lean only, broiled, 4 oz 213
rib chops, with bone, lean only, broiled, 4 oz 239
shoulder, lean only, roasted, boneless, 4 oz 233

Pork
Picnic, without bone and skin, lean only, baked or roasted, 4 oz 239

Veal
loin cuts, lean with fat, braised or broiled, without bone, 4 oz 245
round with rump (roasts and leg cutlets), lean with fat, braised or broiled, without bone, 4 oz 245

Poultry

Chicken
roasted, without skin, 4 oz 204
stewed, light meat without skin, 4 oz 207
Turkey, roasted, light meat without skin, 4 oz 200

101-200 CALORIES

Pasta

All pasta, dry, one cup
cooked till tender, (approx) 190
cooked till firm, (approx) 155

Canned, 1 can

Franco-American macaroni and cheese, 7½ oz	184
Franco-American spaghetti with cheese, 7⅜ oz	170
Franco-American spaghetti with cheese sauce, 7⅜ oz	160

Meat Entrees (at less than 30 calories per ounce)

Frozen

Beef, chipped, creamed	
Banquet, 5 oz	124
Beef, sliced	
Banquet, barbecue sauce, 5 oz	126
Banquet, with gravy, 5 oz	116
Green Giant, 5 oz	130
Beef Stew	
Green Giant Boil-in-Bag, 9 oz	160
Green Giant, with biscuits, 7 oz	190
Veal steaks	
Hormel, 4 oz	130

Meat Entrees, canned (at less than 30 calories per ounce), 1 can

Beef, corned with cabbage
  Hormel, 8 oz 150
Beef stew
  Dinty Moore, 7½ oz 184
  Swanson, 7½ oz 190
Pork, sliced, with gravy
  Morton House, 6¼ oz 190

Poultry entrees

Frozen (at less than 30 calories per ounce)
  Chicken a la King
    Banquet, 5 oz 138
Canned, 1 can
  Chicken stew
    Swanson, 7½ oz 180
  Turkey slices
    Morton House, 6¼ oz 140
  Chicken, fresh
    Broiled, meat only, 4 oz 154

Seafood

Clams, canned, drained, 1 can	
Doxsee, 8 oz	112
Doxsee, 12 oz	147
Shrimp marinara, with shells, frozen	
Buitoni, 4 oz	116

Fish, fresh, 4 oz, meat only

Abalone	111
Black Sea Bass	106
Butterfish, gulf	108
Catfish, fresh water	117
Croaker, Atlantic	109
Lake Herring (Cisco)	109
Lobster	109
Mussels	108
Ocean Pearch, Pacific	108
Red or Grey Snapper	106
Sea bass, white	109
Shrimp	103
Sturgeon	107
Tautog (Blackfish)	101

51-100 CALORIES

Miscellaneous

Pabst Extra Light Beer	70
Whipped butter, 1 Tbsp	65
Farina, *Pillsbury*, ⅔ cup	80
Grits, *Quaker* Instant, 1 packet	79
One Egg, raw or boiled	
extra large	94
large	82
medium	72
Canned Spaghetti with meatballs, *Libby's*, 1 cup	84
Canned Spanish rice, *Libby's*, 1 cup	57

Chinese dishes

Chow mein, canned, 1 cup	
La Choy	
beef	72
chicken	68
mushroom	85
pepper	89
shrimp	61
Chow mein, frozen	
Banquet, 1 bag	89

La Choy beef, 1 cup	97
La Choy shrimp, 1 cup	73
Pea pods, frozen, 1 package	
La Choy	90
Won Ton, frozen, 1 cup	
La Choy	92

Dairy

Cottage Cheese, low fat, ½ cup	
Borden	90
Breakstone	90
Friendship	100
Lucerne	100
Viva	100
Weight Watchers	90
Milk, 8 ounces	
Buttermilk	
.1% fat *Borden*	88
.2% fat *Sealtest* skim	71
.5% fat *Borden*	90
.8% fat *Golden Nugget*	92
.8% fat *Light 'n Lively*	95
Dry, non-fat milk, reconstituted	81
Skin or low-fat	
no fat *Lucerne*	90
.1% fat *Borden*	81

fortified	81
.1% fat *Sealtest*	79
Yogurt, plain, ½ cup	
Borden Lite-Line lowfat	70
Sealtest Light 'n Lively lowfat	70
***Danny On-A-Stick*, uncoated**	65

Meat, canned

Beef stew	
Libby's, 1 cup	78
Ham, whole	
Wilson's certified boned and rolled, 1 oz	56

Poultry

Chicken stew with dumplings, canned	
Libby's, 1 cup	88
Turkey with gravy, frozen	
Banquet, 5 oz	98
Green Giant, 5 oz	100

Seafood, canned

Clams	
Snow's, ½ cup	60
Sau-Sea, 4 oz	99
Gefilte Fish	
Manischewitz, 3 oz piece	53
Manischewitz whitefish and pike, 3 oz piece	64
Mother's, 4 oz piece	55
Oysters	
Bumblebee, ½ cup	86
Shrimp	
Bumblebee, 4½ oz can	90

Seafood, fresh, meat only, 4 oz

Clams	92
Cod	88
Crayfish	82
Croaker, white	95
Flounder	89
Ocean Perch, Atlantic	100
Oysters	75
Pickerel	95
Pike	100
Sand Dab	89
Sauger	95
Scallops	92
Sole	90
Squid	95
Tilefish	90

Fruits and Vegetables

Artichokes
boiled, drained, 1 whole bud 67
Beets
raw, diced, 1 cup 58
Broccoli
boiled, drained, 8 oz 59
Carrots
raw, slices, 1 cup 53
Chayote
raw, 1 medium squash 56
Cranberries
fresh, without stems, 1 cup 52
Currants, red or white
trimmed, 1 cup 55
Dock or Sorrel
raw with stems, 1 lb 89
Endive, French or Belgian
trimmed, 1 lb 68
Escarole
untrimmed, 1 lb 80
Grapefruit
pink or red, with seeds
whole, with skin, 1 lb 87
sections, 1 cup 80
pink or red, seedless
whole, with skin, 1 lb 93
sections, 1 cup 80

Food	Calories
white, with seeds	
whole, with skin, 1 lb	84
sections, 1 cup	82
white, seedless	
whole, with skin, 1 lb	87
sections, 1 cup	78
Honeydew Melon	
whole, with rinds and seeds, 1 lb	94
cubed or diced, 1 cup	56
Lettuce	
Iceberg	
whole, 1 lb	56
Loose Leaf	
whole, 1 lb	52
Romaine or cos	
whole, 1 lb	52
Pawpaw	
peeled and seeded, 4 oz	96
Papaya	
peeled and seeded, cubed, 1 cup	55
Peaches	
pared, sliced, 1 cup	65
Raspberries	
black, 1 cup	98
red, 1 cup	70
Strawberries	
whole, 1 cup	55
Watermelon	
whole, with rind, 1 lb	54

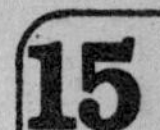

20-50 CALORIES

Breads, Buns and Rolls

Bread, 1 slice	
Gluten	
Thomas	32
Protein	
Thomas	45
Rice Cakes	
Spiral	36
Wheat	
Thomas	50
White	
Arnold Melba Thin	40
Fresh Horizons	50
Pepperidge Farm Very Thin	40
Weight Watchers	35
Buns and Rolls, 1 piece	
Pepperidge Farm Old-Fashioned	37
Pepperidge Farm Party	35
Margarine, 1 Tbsp	
Blue Bonnet Diet	50
Fleischmann Diet	50
Imitation	50

Candy, 1 piece

Rolo 28

Cheese, 1 oz

Farmer's
Friendship 38
Ricotta
Borden 42
Imitation Cream Cheese
Philadelphia 50
American, grated
Borden 30

Chinese Dishes

Apple-Cinnamon roll, frozen
La Choy, 1 piece 38
Bamboo Shoots, canned
La Choy, 8 oz 23
Bean sprouts, canned
La Choy, 8 oz 24
Chow Mein, canned, 1 cup
Chun King 44
La Choy, meatless 47

Egg Rolls, frozen	
La Choy chicken, 1 piece	30
La Choy lobster, 1 piece	27
Mixed vegetables, canned	
La Choy, 1 cup	35

Cream

Half & Half, 1 Tbsp	20
Lucerne Real Cream topping, 1 whipped oz	20

Dips, 1 oz

Bean, Jalapeño	
Frito-Lay	36
Gebhardt	30
Granny Goose	37
Lucerne	36
Clam	
Lucerne	34
Gelatin	
Knox gelatin, 1 envelope	28
Gravy	
French's Pork, mix, ½ cup	40

Jelly, 1 Tbsp

Apple	
Kraft, Low Calorie	22
Diet Delight	22
Apricot Pineapple Jam	
Diet Delight	21
Blackberry Apple	
Kraft, low calorie	22
Blackberry Jam	
Diet Delight	21
Grape	
Kraft, Low Calorie	22
Diet Delight	21
Raspberry Jam	
Diet Delight	21

Meat, 1 oz, canned

Beef	
Corned, canned	
Safeway	35
Dried	
Swift	42
Smoked	
Safeway	35
Safeway spicy	40

Beef roast	
Wilson	33
Ham	
Wilson certified fully cooked	48
Wilson certified *Tender Made*	44
Wilson certified festival ham	48
Pastrami	
Safeway	40
Scrapple	
Oscar Mayer in tube	50
Oscar Mayer Philadelphia style	45

Olives

Green, 10 large	**45**
Manzanillo Black, 10 large	**50**

Popcorn, 1 cup

***Pops-Rite*, popped**	**38**
***Wise*, cheese-flavored, ready to eat**	**49**

Poultry

Safeway smoked chicken, 1 oz	50
Safeway smoked turkey, 1 oz	50

Pudding, ½ cup

D-Zerta	
butterscotch	25
chocolate	20
vanilla	30

Salad Dressing, 1 Tbsp

French	
Ann Page Low Calorie	25
Kraft Low Calorie	25
Nu Made Low Calorie	20
Italian	
Wish-Bone Low Calorie	20
May Lo Naise	
Tillie Lewis	25
Russian	
Wish-Bone Low Calorie	25

Thousand Island	
Ann Page Low Calorie	25
Wish-Bone Low Calorie	25
Whipped	
Tillie Lewis	25

Sauces & Spreads

Crosse & Blackwell Anchovy Paste 1 Tbsp	20
***Hunt's* Tomato Sauce, 4 oz**	35
with mushrooms, 4 oz	40
***Open Pit* Barbecue, 1 Tbsp**	26

Vegetables, canned and frozen

Artichoke Hearts	
Birds Eye, 3 oz	20
Asparagus, 1 cup, canned	
cuts	40
spears	40
spears and tips	35
whole	50
Asparagus, frozen	
Birds Eye, 3.3 oz	25
Seabrook Farms, ½ cup	23

Beans, green canned, 1 cup	
french	
Del Monte	40
Green Giant	30
Kounty Kist	40
Libby's	35
whole	
Del Monte	35
Green Giant	30
Kounty Kist	40
Libby's	35
Stokely-Van Camp	40
Beans, green, frozen	
Birds Eye, 3.3 oz	25
Kounty Kist, 1 cup	30
Seabrook Farms, 1 cup	42
Beans, wax or yellow, 1 cup	
Del Monte	35
Libby's	40
Stokely-Van Camp	45
Broccoli, frozen	
Birds Eye 3.3 oz	25
Green Giant, 1 cup	30
Kounty Kist, 1 cup	30
Seabrook Farms, 1 cup	46
Brussels Sprouts, frozen	
Birds Eye, 3.3 oz	30
Green Giant, 1 cup	50
Kounty Kist, 1 cup	50

Carrots, canned, 1 cup	
Libby's	40
S & W	44
Cauliflower, frozen	
Birds Eye 3.3 oz	25
Green Giant, 1 cup	25
Kounty Kist, 1 cup	25
Collard Greens	
Birds Eye, 3.3 oz	30
Seabrook Farms, 1 cup	44
Mixed Vegetables	
Kounty Kist, California, 1 cup	30
Mustard Greens	
Seabrook Farms, ½ cup	21
Sauerkraut, canned, 1 cup	50
Spinach, canned, 1 cup	45
Spinach, frozen, 1 cup	50
Tomatoes, canned	
Hunt's stewed, 4 oz	30
Libby's whole, 1 cup	45
S & W whole, 1 cup	42
Stokely-Van Camp, whole	50
Townhouse, whole	50
Turnip Greens	
Birds Eye 3.3 oz	20
Seabrook Farms, ½ cup	22
Stokely-Van Camp, ½ cup	22

Fruits and Vegetables, fresh, 1 cup unless noted

Asparagus	
cut spears	35
Bamboo shoots	
cuts	41
Bean Sprouts	37
Beans, green or snap	
cuts	34
Beans, wax or yellow	
cuts	30
Beet Greens	26
Cabbage, red or green, chopped	22
Cantelope, cubed	48
Casaba Melon, cubed	45
Cauliflower, flowerets	27
Swiss Chard, leaves only	32
Eggplant, diced	50
Radish, diced	20
Rhubarb, raw diced	20
Summer Squash, diced	35
Tomatos, sliced	40
Turnips, cubed	39

Fruit and Vegetable drinks, 6 oz

Cranberry	
Ocean Spray low calorie	35

Cranberry apple	
Ocean Spray cranapple low calorie	30
Sauerkraut	
Libby's	20
Tomato	
Campbell's	35
Del Monte	35
Heinz	38
Hunt's	43
Libby's	39
S & W	22
Sacramento	35
Stokely-Van Camp	33
Townhouse	35
Welch's	38
Tomato cocktail	
Ortega Snap-E-Tom	38
Vegetable cocktail	
S & W	21
Townhouse	35
V-8	35

UNDER 20 CALORIES

Beverages

Note: virtually all sodas that are called *low-calorie*, *sugar-free* or *dietetic* contain 2 calories or less.

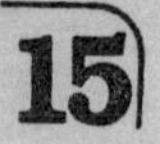

Bouillon, 1 cube

Beef	
Herb-Ox	6
Maggi	6
Wyler's	7
Wyler's Instant	10
Chicken	
Herb-Ox	6
Maggi	7
Wyler's	8
Wyler's Instant	6
Onion	
Herb-Ox	10
Wyler's	6
Vegetable	
Herb-Ox	6
Wyler's	6

Breath Mints, 1 piece

Certs **clear**	8
Certs **pressed**	6
Chewels	10
Clorets **mints**	6
Dentyne **dynamints**	2
Lifesavers	7
Trident **mints**	8

Broth, 1 packet

Herb-Ox	
Beef	8
Chicken	12
Onion	14
Vegetable	12

Candy, Dietetic

***Estee*, 1 piece**	
chocolate covered raisins	**6**
gum drops	**3**
hard candies	**12**
mint candies	**4**

Cocktail Mix, non-alcoholic, 1 oz

***Holland House* Bloody Mary**	**6**
***Holland House* Whiskey Sour**	**9**

Coffee, 1 cup

ground	**2**
instant	**4**

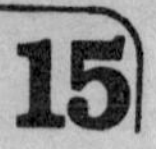

Condiments, 1 Tbsp

A-*1* sauce	12
Catsup	
Del Monte	15
Chili sauce	
Heinz	17
Horseradish	2
Mustard	
French's Brown	15
French's Yellow	16
Grey Poupon Dijon	15
Soy sauce	
La Choy	8
Taco sauce	
Old El Paso	4
Vinegar	1
Worcestershire	10

Cookies, 1 piece

Angel Puffs	
Stella D'Oro Dietetic	17
Arrowroot	
Sunshine	16
Royal Nuggets	
Stella D'Oro	1

Vanilla Snaps
Nabisco 13
Vanilla Wafers
Sunshine 15
Nabisco 18
Zuzu Ginger Snaps
Nabisco 16

Cough Drops 9

Crackers, 1 cracker

Cheez-It
Sunshine 6
Cheeze
Keebler 11
Flings Curls
Nabisco 10
Matzos
Manischewitz Tam Tams 14
Melba Toast
Old London
Garlic 9
Onion 10
Pumpernickel 17
Rye 17
Sesame 10
Wheat 17
White 17

Oyster	
Keebler	3
Sunshine	3
Ritz	
Nabisco	16
Saltines	
Keebler Zesta	12
Nabisco Premium	12
Sunshine Krispy	11
Sociables	
Nabisco	10
Triangle Thins	
Nabisco	8
Wheat Thins	
Nabisco	9

Creamers, Non-Dairy, 1 tsp

Coffee-Mate, Carnation, 1 pkt	11
Coffee-Tone	12
Cremora, Pet	11

Gelatin, mix, ½ cup

D-Zerta	8
Royal Sweet As You Please	6

Gravy, ¼ cup, mix

Au Jus	
Durkee	8
French's	8
McCormick	4
Schilling	4
Brown	
Durkee	15
Durkee with mushrooms	15
Durkee with onions	17
McCormick Lite	10
Weight Watchers	8
with mushrooms	12
with onions	13
Chicken	
Durkee home style	18
McCormick Lite	10
Pillsbury home style	15
Schilling Lite	10
Weight Watchers	10
Mushroom	
McCormick	19
Schilling	19
Pork	
Durkee	18
Mushroom Steak	
Dawn Fresh	4
Swiss Steak	
Durkee	11

Gum, 1 piece

Adams	9
Beeman	10
Beech-Nut	9
Beechies	6
Black Jack	9
Care Free	8
Chiclets	6
Clorets	6
Clove	5
Dentyne	5
Estee	3
Freshen-Up	9
Fruit Stripe	9
Orbit	8
Trident	5
Wrigley's	10

Jelly, 1 tsp

Ann Page, all flavors	18
Diet Delight Strawberry	18
Kraft, all flavors	16
S & W, all flavors	10
Smuckers Slenderella, all flavors	8

Oil

Pam Vegetable spray	7

Pickles

Capers, 1 Tbsp	
Crosse & Blackwell	6
Onions, cocktail, 1 Tbsp	
Crosse & Blackwell	1
Peppers, 1 oz	
Chile Green, *Ortega*	5
Hot Pickled, *Old El Paso*	9
Dill Pickles, spears, 1 piece	
Bond's	2
Del Monte	7
Heinz	7
Smucker's	8
Sour Pickles, 1 piece	
Del Monte	10

Salad dressings, 1 Tbsp

Blue Cheese	
Ann Page Low Calorie	18
Kraft Low Calorie	14

Tillie Lewis	12
Weight Watchers	10
Caesar	
Pfeiffer Low Calorie	10
French	
Pfeiffer Low Calorie	18
Weight Watchers	4
Tillie Lewis	12
Italian	
Ann Page Low Calorie	14
Kraft Low Calorie	6
Nu Made Low Calorie	16
Pfeiffer Low Calorie	10
Tillie Lewis	6
Weight Watchers	2
Red Wine	
Pfeiffer Low Calorie	10
Russian	
Pfeiffer Low Calorie	15
Tillie Lewis	12
Weight Watchers	12
Thousand Island	
Pfeiffer Low Calorie	15
Tillie Lewis	18
Weight Watchers	12

Sauces, 1 Tbsp

Barbecue	
French's	14
Enchilada	
Old El Paso hot	9
Old El Paso mild	10
Lemon-Butter	
Weight Watchers	8

Sugar, 1 tsp — 15

Pancake Syrup, 1 Tbsp

Cary's Diet	10
Diet Delight	15
S & W	12
Tillie Lewis	14

Tea, 1 cup — 1

lemon-flavored	
Nestea	2

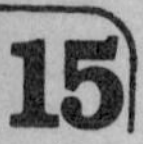

Toppings, 1 Tbsp

No-Cal	
all flavors except chocolate and coffee	0
No-Cal chocolate & coffee	6
whipped mix	
D-Zerta	8
Dream Whip	10

Vegetables and Fruits, Fresh

Cabbage	
Chinese, cuts, 1 cup	11
spoon (Bakchoy), cuts, 1 cup	11
Celery	
1 large outer stalk	7
3 small inner stalks	9
Chicory greens	
cuts, 1 cup	11
10 inner leaves	5
Endive, French or Belgian	
1 head, 5-7"	8
10 small leaves	5
chopped, 1 cup	14
Escarole, cuts, 1 cup	10
Mushrooms, chopped, 1 cup	20
Pepper, sweet, green, sliced, 1 cup	18

Pickles	
dill, 1 large	15
sour, 1 large	14
Spinach, trimmed and chopped, 1 cup	14
Watercress, 1 cup	7